Mosby's

Pharmacy
Technician

LAB MANUAL

Mosby's

Pharmacy Technician
LAB MANUAL

JUDITH L. NEVILLE

Pharmacy Technician Program Director/
Externship Coordinator

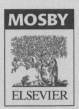

MOSBY
ELSEVIER

3251 Riverport Lane
Maryland Heights, MO 63043

MOSBY'S PHARMACY TECHNICIAN LAB MANUAL,
FIRST EDITION REVISED REPRINT
ISBN 13: 978-0-323-08812-1

ISBN 13: 978-0-323-08812-1

Publishing Director: *Andrew Allen*
Executive Editor: *Jennifer Janson*
Developmental Editor: *Kelly Brinkman*
Publishing Services Manager: *Julie Eddy*
Senior Project Manager: *Rich Barber*
Designer: *Andrea Lutes*

Printed in the United States

Last digit is the print number: 9   8   7   6   5   4   3   2

Preface

Welcome to the exciting world of Pharmacy Technology! You have started on a journey into one of today's fastest-growing fields in health care. Whether you will end up working in a hospital pharmacy, a community pharmacy, one of the large pharmacy chain stores, or another location, the knowledge you will gain from this lab manual will help prepare you well for your new career.

Pharmacy technicians are increasingly called upon to perform duties traditionally fulfilled by pharmacists. This is because of new federal regulations that now require pharmacists to spend more time with patients providing patient education. Because of the nature of the pharmacy technician's work, hands-on training is critically important in educational programs. This lab manual is designed to provide hands-on training and help you master the information and skills necessary to be a successful pharmacy technician. The various labs will challenge your knowledge, help further reinforce key concepts, and allow you to gauge your understanding of the subject matter that you have studied in your pharmacy technician program.

Mosby's Pharmacy Technician Lab Manual is a reliable and understandable resource written specifically for the pharmacy technician student and for those technicians already on the job who are preparing for the National Pharmacy Technician Certification exam (PCTB), or the Certified Pharmacy Technician exam (CPhT). The content of the lab manual is written so that it may easily accompany Hopper: *Mosby's Pharmacy Technician: Principles & Practice*. The manual is divided into eight sections—Retail Ambulatory Pharmacy, Inpatient Pharmacy, Extemporaneous Compounding, Aseptic Technique and IV Compounding, Communication in the Pharmacy, Ethics and Law, Essential Technician Skills and Drug Product Knowledge, and Pharmacy Office.

The Evolve Companion website offers a resource that allows both instructors and students to harness the power of the World Wide Web. An English/Spanish audio glossary and list of common pharmacy abbreviations provide students with additional information needed for success. Instructors can access an Instructor's Manual, Lab Notes, and a 150-question test bank, as well as the student Evolve materials, through Evolve at http://evolve.elsevier.com.

Contents

UNIT 1 **Retail Ambulatory Pharmacy**
LAB 1:   Orientation to the Retail Lab, 3
LAB 2:   Hand Hygiene, 5
LAB 3:   Counting Oral Medication, 7
LAB 4:   Prescription Interpretation, 9
LAB 5:   Insurance Cards, 13
LAB 6:   Data Entry, 16
LAB 7:   Processing Retail Prescriptions, 19
LAB 8:   Refilling a Retail Prescription, 22
LAB 9:   Refill Data Entry, 27
LAB 10:   Home Medical Equipment, 30
LAB 11:   Glucose Monitor, 34
LAB 12:   Automated Dispensing Systems: Baker Cells, 37
LAB 13:   Health Insurance Portability and Accountability Act (HIPAA), 41
LAB 14:   Mail Order, 46

UNIT 2 **Inpatient Pharmacy**
LAB 15:   Processing Inpatient Prescriptions, 55
LAB 16:   Automation, 60

UNIT 3 **Extemporaneous Compounding**
LAB 17, part I: Balance, 65
LAB 17, part II: Compounding, 68
LAB 17, part III: Compounding, 71
LAB 17, part IV: Compounding, 75

UNIT 4 **Aseptic Technique and IV Compounding**
LAB 18:   Introduction to Aseptic IV Compounding Pharmacy, 81
LAB 19, part I: Aseptic Technique, 84
LAB 19, part II: Aseptic Technique, 87
LAB 20:   Cleaning a Horizontal Laminar Airflow Hood, 90
LAB 21:   Horizontal Laminar Airflow Hood, 93
LAB 22:   Cleaning the Vertical Airflow Hood, 95

LAB 23:   Withdrawing Medication from a Vial, 97
LAB 24:   Withdrawing Medication from an Ampule, 101
LAB 25:   Reconstituting Dry Powder, 105
LAB 26:   Introducing Liquid into an IV Bag, 108
LAB 27:   Hazardous Drugs, 112

UNIT 5 **Communication in the Pharmacy**
LAB 28, part I: Nonverbal Communication, 119
LAB 28, part II: Communication Skills, 121
LAB 28, part III: Communication, 124
LAB 29:   Spanish for the Pharmacy Technician, 127

UNIT 6 **Ethics and Law**
LAB 30:   Ethics, 135
LAB 31:   Law, 140

UNIT 7 **Essential Technician Skills and Drug Product Knowledge**
LAB 32:   Over-the-Counter Labels, 145
LAB 33:   Design a Drug, 149
LAB 34:   Controlled Drugs, 158
LAB 35:   Brand-Generic, 163
LAB 36:   Medication Errors, 166
LAB 37:   Advanced Prescription Interpretation, 169
LAB 38:   Reference Materials, 171
LAB 39:   Conversions, 176

UNIT 8 **Pharmacy Office**
LAB 40:   Reports: Inventory Management, 181
LAB 41:   Business Math, 183
LAB 42:   Prior Authorizations, 185
LAB 43:   Medicare, 190

Bibliography, 193

Retail Ambulatory Pharmacy

Orientation to the Retail Lab

OBJECTIVE

- Identify and become familiar with pharmacy supplies and equipment.

Pre-Lab Experience

1. Visit the following website: *www.pharmex.com*.
2. Select *Pharmacy Warning Labels* from the column on the left of the screen.
   An *auxiliary label* provides additional instructions to the patient.
   A *warning label* alerts the patient to specific warnings on administration and storage of the medication, as well as potential food and drug interactions.

ORIENTATION TO THE RETAIL LAB

1. Locate the following items in the retail lab:
   a. Counting trays
   b. Wooden-handled counting spatula
   c. Amber vials
   d. Stock medication bottles
   e. Auxiliary/warning labels
   f. Graduated cylinder
   g. Ovals or ointment jars
   h. Quick-grab medications

2. Choose an auxiliary label and affix it in the space provided.

3. Choose a warning auxiliary label and affix it in the space provided.

4. How are the stock medication bottles arranged?

5. What is the maximum amount in milliliters that the graduated cylinder will measure?

6. What does the acronym *POS* stand for? Describe where this is located in the retail pharmacy lab.

Student Name _____ Date _____

Lab Partner _____

Grade/Comments _____

_____

Student Comments _____

_____

Hand Hygiene

OBJECTIVES

- Demonstrate effective hand-washing technique.

- Identify the benefits of effective hand hygiene.

Pre-Lab Experience

Read an overview of the guidelines for hand hygiene in health care settings. Make special note of the definitions and techniques of hand hygiene. A PowerPoint presentation can be found at *www.cdc.gov/ handhygiene/download/hand_hygiene_core.ppt.*

The presentation also can be found by following these steps:

1. Web address: *www.cdc.gov/*
2. Type in hand hygiene in the search box.
3. View the PowerPoint presentation "Hand Hygiene in Healthcare Settings Core."

HAND HYGIENE

The most important means of preventing the spread of infection is frequent and effective hand washing. Hands must be washed using the correct technique. The first scrub of the morning should be extensive, lasting 2 to 4 minutes. An antimicrobial soap with antiseptic residual action that will last several hours should be used.

Proper hand washing requires running water and friction. The water should be warm, because water that is too cold or too hot will cause skin chapping. Friction involves firmly rubbing all surfaces of the hands and wrists.

Demonstrate the following:

☐ Using soap and warm and running water, firmly rub hands together using an antimicrobial soap.
☐ Thoroughly wash palms, back of hands, fingers, under the fingernails, and wrists. Do this for at least 10 to 15 seconds.
☐ Rinse hands thoroughly. Allow water to run off the fingertips.
☐ Dry hands using a clean paper towel. Pat your skin dry rather than rubbing to avoid chapping.
☐ Turn off the water using the towel (not your bare hands).

QUESTIONS FOR REVIEW

1. Does proper hand washing sterilize your skin? Explain.

2. What two factors does proper hand washing require?

Student Name _____ Date _____

Lab Partner _____

Grade/Comments _____

_____

Student Comments _____

_____

Counting Oral Medication

OBJECTIVES

- Demonstrate the ability to count oral medication manually.

- Become familiar with cleaning procedures within the pharmacy setting.

Pre-Lab Information

Isopropyl alcohol (70%) serves as a general cleaner and disinfectant for the pharmacy area. General cleaning of counting trays, counting spatulas, and work surface areas will be a routine task for a pharmacy technician. Cleaning with soap and water removes dirt and most germs. However, disinfecting provides an extra margin of safety.

PART ONE

A. Counting oral medication
1. Prepare a work area for yourself on the counter that is free from clutter.
2. Place a *clean* counting tray and counting spatula on the counter in front of you.
3. Choose a stock bottle of oral medication from the shelf.
4. Dump or pour a partial amount of tablets from the stock bottle onto your counting tray.

5. Open the lid on the "pour" compartment or well of your tray.
6. Using your spatula, begin counting the tablets in increments of five.
7. As you count the tablets, slide them into the pour compartment or well of your tray.
8. Continue counting by fives until you have reached the desired number of tablets needed.
9. You may need to pour additional tablets from the stock bottle onto your tray.
10. When you have finished counting, close the tray lid.
11. Return any unused tablets to the stock bottle.
12. Securely replace the lid on the stock bottle.
13. Select an amber vial and place the vial beside the counting tray.
14. Pour the counted tablets into the vial.
15. Place a lid on the vial.

B. Practice counting the following quantities. Indicate with a checkmark when task is complete.

    #30 _____

    #15 _____

    #60 _____

C. Replace stock bottles and all other supplies when counting exercise is completed. *The lab is not complete until materials used are replaced on the appropriate shelf.*

PART TWO

Clean the counting tray and counting spatula by using the premixed solution of isopropyl alcohol and water. This is done by spraying the disinfectant solution on the counting equipment and then using a paper towel to clean.

Use this same disinfectant solution periodically to clean the work surfaces in the pharmacy lab.

Student Name _____ Date _____

Lab Partner _____

Grade/Comments _____

_____

Student Comments _____

_____

Prescription Interpretation

OBJECTIVE

- Identify necessary information needed on a retail prescription.

Pre-Lab Information

Prescriptions often are referred to as scripts. Script means to write, to scribble.

PRESCRIPTION INTERPRETATION

Pharmacy technicians accept written prescription orders from patients daily. The technician is responsible for performing an overview of the prescription in order to check for completeness. The pharmacy technician also must check for accurate prescription information.

Directions

Interpret the following outpatient prescriptions. Answer the questions corresponding with each script.

Dr. Mark Paulsen   office: 800/777-2211
2100 Lake Avenue
Farmview, IA 51223

Patient Name__Andrea Lawler_____   Date__3/7/07_____
Address_____

        Refill____0____Times

        Rx: Indocin 25mg BID pc
            #30

Dr. Mark Paulsen
_____
Product Selection Permitted   **Dispense As Written**

DEA NO._____
Address_____

1. What is the drug that should be dispensed?

2. May a generic equivalent be dispensed on this prescription?

3. What are the directions to the patient in lay terms?

Dr. Mark Paulsen   office: 800/777-2211
2100 Lake Avenue
Farmview, IA 51223

Patient Name___Gloria Stimes_____   Date _4/12/07_____
Address_____
                                        Refill____1___Times

        Rx: Glucophage 500mg
            #60
         Sig: BID

Dr. Mark Paulsen
_____
Product Selection Permitted   **Dispense As Written**

DEA NO._____
Address_____

1. Are there refills allowed on this prescription?

2. What are the directions to the patient in lay terms?

3. What is the name and dosage of medication to be dispensed?

4. How many tablets will be dispensed?

Dr. Mark Paulsen   office: 800/777-2211
2100 Lake Avenue
Farmview, IA 51223

> Patient Name____Carl Jarlton_____
> Date__3/21/07_____
> Address__109 7th. St._____
>
> Refill__0_____Times
>
> Rx: Duragestic Patch 50mcg/hr
> #5
> Sig: Apply patch q 72 hr.

Dr. Mark Paulsen

Product Selection Permitted   **Dispense As Written**

DEA NO._AP1372321_____
Address_____

---

1. Is the patient allowed any refills on this prescription?

2. Is the patient's address necessary on this prescription? Why or why not?

3. Is the physician's DEA number necessary on this prescription? Why or why not?

4. What is the medication name and dosage to be dispensed?

5. What are the instructions to the patient?

COUNTING RECORD

Student Name: _____

Directions

The purpose of this exercise is to increase accuracy and speed in counting oral medication. Work with a lab partner when practicing in the lab. On the chart, indicate the date of your counting lab. Your partner will initial the appropriate date to indicate that he or she has observed you counting.

Date						
Student Initials						
Date						
Partner Initials						

Student Name _____ Date _____

Lab Partner _____

Grade/Comments _____

_____

Student Comments _____

_____

Insurance Cards

OBJECTIVES

- Summarize patient information needed to process a prescription insurance claim.

- Become aware of common reasons for denial of insurance claims.

Pre-Lab Information

Prescription drug discount cards tie in closely with insurance identification cards. Just like insurance cards, prescription drug discount cards allow patients to save money on all types of prescription medications. At the time of purchase the patient will present the card to receive discounts instantly on the prescription drugs. Familiarity with the discount drug companies with which the pharmacy participates will be beneficial for the pharmacy technician.

INSURANCE CARDS

To process claims, the technician must be able to obtain all the information that is needed to process that claim. The patient will present an insurance identification card at the time of prescription drop-off. Personal identification information and insurance information are provided on the identification card.

Personal information includes the following:

1. Full legal name
2. Date of birth (DOB)
3. Address

Insurance information includes the following:

1. Name of the insurance company
2. Prescription carrier name
3. Identification (ID) number
4. Group number
5. Person number
6. Dependent number

This information allows the insurance prescription carrier to process the claim electronically and send back a response of paid or denied to the pharmacy immediately.

This information also allows the carrier to send the retail pharmacy a price to charge the customer. The customer charge may be a percentage of the price of the prescription or may be a flat co-payment. The customer may pay full price for the prescription because there could be a deductible to meet before the carrier picks up prescription costs. The patient may have no charge for the prescription if the insurance carrier pays the full amount.

Each insurance plan is different, as are the insurance cards. Pharmacy technicians should become familiar with insurance cards and should be able to recognize each card.

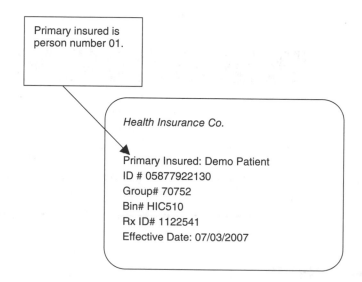

At the time of prescription drop-off, ask the patient whether he or she is the primary card holder.

Primary is the card holder known as 01 or 00. Input the correct card holder code in the computer. The spouse of the cardholder is 02. Children are coded 03 for the oldest child, 04 for the middle child, and so on.

ACTIVITY

Student Directions

Compare personal insurance cards with a lab partner. Locate the personal identification information and the information contained on the reverse side of the card. (Ask your instructor for sample insurance/discount drug cards if you prefer not to share your personal card.)

1. List five important items found on the front of an insurance card.

2. What information is found on the back side of the insurance card?

Rejection Claims

After submitting a claim, rejection messages may be returned. The pharmacy technician is responsible for finding out why the claim was rejected. The technician may call the insurance company help desk to help decipher the rejection claim. The help desk phone number is located on the reverse side of the insurance identification card. The help desk specialist and the pharmacy technician will compare patient information in order to resolve the claim rejection.

Reasons for claim rejection may be the following:

- Invalid person code
- Invalid DOB
- Dependent exceeds age limit
- Invalid gender
- Prescriber is not network provider
- Unable to connect
- Patient not covered
- Refill too soon
- Refills not covered
- NDC not covered

Student Name _____ Date _____

Lab Partner _____

Grade/Comments _____

_____

Student Comments _____

_____

Data Entry

OBJECTIVES

- Perform necessary computer functions to enter a new prescription into a pharmacy-specific software system.

- Demonstrate the ability to navigate through a pharmacy-specific software system.

Pre-Lab Information

Please review these basic terms and directions in order to better understand the pharmacy software program used in the data entry labs, Visual SuperScript:

Clicking—clicking the left mouse button once to select option

Icons—buttons with pictures on them that will indicate the purpose of the icon

Screen tip—brief description of the function of the icon that appears by moving the mouse pointer to the icon and leaving it on the icon for a few seconds

Text boxes—data entry areas or fields used to input information; some of these areas/fields may have drop-down lists for predetermined entries

Blinking cursor—provides a visual cue as to which item is currently selected

Tab key—the key to use to move between fields/areas on the screen forms. Do not use the enter key!

F3—function key located at the top of your keyboard that allows for more detailed information. First, select the menu item, and then press the F3 key.

Edit boxes—data entry areas where large amounts of text may be entered

NOTE: Each menu item may be selected by clicking on it with the mouse OR by pressing the *Alt* key and the corresponding underlined letter for each menu choice. Software is not included with this manual.

DATA ENTRY: ENTERING A NEW PRESCRIPTION

Regardless of the practice setting for the pharmacy technician, entering data into the computer is a major component of the workload. In the retail setting, for instance, a customer drops off the prescription hard copy. After the technician has obtained all the necessary information from the customer, the technician enters the information into the computer. This lab explains the steps involved in filling new prescriptions and refilling existing ones.

Use the following prescription for the lab exercise.

Dr. John Thompson   office: 800/777-2211
2100 Lake Avenue
Farmview, IA 51223

Patient Name__Karen Anderson   **Date**__3/7/07_____
Address_____

          Refill_____2_____Times

          Rx: Lipitor 10mg
                i q hs
          #30

                                        Dr. John Thompson

Product Selection Permitted   **Dispense As Written**

DEA NO._____
Address_____

---

1. Place the *Visual SuperScript* CD into your computer.
2. Enter your password and select *Fill Rx's* on the menu screen.
3. Click on the *New Rx* icon on the top left of the screen.
4. Prescription information such as the prescription number and dispense date is generated automatically and added to the form. Highlight the text in the *RPh* text box by using your mouse.
5. You then will be prompted to the *Customer's Name* text box.
6. Press the *F3* key to bring up the customer database/pick list.
7. Select *Karen Anderson* as your customer by double-clicking on her name.
8. Change the RPh initials to your first initial and then *tech.* For example, Tom would be TTECH. Change the prescription date, if needed.
9. Karen Anderson's personal information, such as her address and phone number, will be added automatically to the fill screen.
10. Press the *Tab* key. You then will be prompted to the *Doctor* text box.
11. Select John Thompson as the prescribing doctor.
12. Press the *Tab* key. You will be prompted to the *Prescribed Drug* text box.
13. Karen Anderson's prescription is for Lipitor 10 mg. Type the first three letters of the drug into the text box "Lip" and then press *Enter*.

14. A pick list will appear. Select Lipitor 10-mg tablet from the pick list by double-clicking on the drug name.
15. A series of warning dialog boxes will appear. Click on *Continue Rx* to navigate to the next step.
16. Double-click on the drug name a second time. The drug information such as NDC and manufacturer will be added automatically to the fill screen.
17. Next, you will be prompted to the *Refills Ordered* text box. Karen Anderson has two refills on this prescription. Type "2" in the text box.
18. Press the *Tab* key. You will be prompted to enter the prescribed quantity. Karen Anderson's prescription is for 30 tablets.
19. Press the *Tab* key until you reach the *DAW* text box. Choose number *1: Physician DAW* from the DAW (dispense as written) list box. Do this by clicking on the arrow on the right side of the list box. A submenu will appear. Click on *1: Physician DAW*.
20. Press the *Tab* key. Enter directions for using the drug in the *Sig* text box. The prescription for Karen Anderson is for one tablet every evening. If an error is made when typing the sig, use your mouse to highlight the error and retype the correct information.
21. Press the *Tab* key. You will be prompted to enter *Prescribed Days Supply*. Type in "1" for Karen Anderson's day's supply.
22. Press the *Tab* key. You are now prompted to save the prescription information.
23. Answer the following questions.

NEW PRESCRIPTION DATA ENTRY

1. How is the entry field identified?

2. What procedure do you follow to look up a new patient in the system?

3. What keyboard character separates the patient's last name from the first name?

4. Are you able to use shorthand when entering new prescription information? Explain by giving an example.

5. Click on the *Insurance Plan* tab on the fill screen for Karen Anderson. What is the plan name and company of Karen Anderson's insurance?

Student Name _____ Date _____

Lab Partner _____

Grade/Comments _____

_____

Student Comments _____

_____

Processing Retail Prescriptions

OBJECTIVE

- Demonstrate the process of filling a prescription in the retail setting.

Pre-Lab Information

The pharmacy technician is responsible for gathering pertinent information from customers when prescriptions are dropped off at the retail counter. The pharmacy technician must communicate effectively by using a clear voice and by using appropriate body language. Eye contact with the customer shows your interest and concern.

OTC: over the counter

PROCESSING A RETAIL PRESCRIPTION

The prescription order is part of the professional relationship among the prescriber, the pharmacy team, and the patient. The pharmacy is responsible for providing quality care that meets the medication needs of the patient.

Demonstrate the following steps:

1. Receive the prescription.
   a. Ask patient for pertinent information.
       i. DOB
      ii. Full name
     iii. Payment source (insurance, cash)

        iv. Allergies

        v. Other medications patient may be taking (include OTC vitamins, herbals, and other products)

    b. *Check* that the prescription is complete and accurate (date, signature of physician, medication name, dose and strength, full patient name).

2. Translate the prescription.
   a. Read through entire prescription.
      i. Are the directions clear?
3. Enter the information into the computer system.
   a. Compare and *check* computer-generated label with the hard copy.
   b. Make sure patient directions are clear and easy to understand.
4. Fill the prescription order.
   a. Take the computer-generated label to the shelf and locate correct stock bottle.
   b. Compare and *check* stock bottle NDC with label NDC.
   c. Return to work area and count medication.
   d. Transfer counted drug to the appropriate vial.
      i. Be certain to use appropriate lid.
   e. *Check* medication dispensed against label.
   f. Place an X on stock bottle for inventory purposes.
   g. Initial the label.
   h. Apply label to vial. Apply second part of label to the back side of the hard copy.
   i. Apply auxiliary labels.
   j. Place vial, stock bottle, and original script together for pharmacist's *check*.
5. Notify pharmacist that medication is ready to be checked.
6. After pharmacist has checked the medication, proceed to POS area.
   a. Distribute HIPAA information.
   b. Notify the patient that counseling is available through the pharmacist.
   c. Complete transaction.
7. Pharmacist will counsel.
8. Return stock medication bottles to shelves.
9. File hard copy.

QUESTIONS FOR REVIEW

1. How many checks should the pharmacy technician make when processing a medication order? Explain.

2. Who are four persons to consult if you are unsure of the drug name on the prescription order?

3. What is the procedure when asking another team member to decipher a drug order?

Student Name _____ Date _____

Lab Partner _____

Grade/Comments _____

_____

Student Comments _____

_____

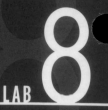

Refilling a Retail Prescription

OBJECTIVE

• Indicate the steps involved in refilling a prescription.

Pre-Lab Information

It is important to note that controlled medications have refill restrictions that are more stringent than those of other legend drugs. Although pharmacy rules and regulations vary from state to state, follow these general guidelines:

• Any controlled drug listed in schedule II is not allowed any refills.
• Any prescription for a controlled substance listed in schedules III to V shall be refilled no more than 6 months after the date on which the prescription was issued and can be refilled no more than 5 times.

Learn more about the refill laws in your state. Use the Internet to access your state pharmacy rules and regulations regarding refills for controlled drugs: *www.statelocalgov.net/*

Search the site for your state pharmacy board, for example, Nebraska Board of Pharmacy.

REFILLS

When processing a refill prescription, be sure to check that there are refills available. Most pharmacy computer programs allow looking up a refill by prescription number or through the patient profile. The computer screen will indicate when no refills are available.

Follow these steps if there are no refills for the medication:

- Alert the customer. The customer possibly may have a new prescription for the medication.
- Alert the pharmacist.
- Depending on your pharmacy procedure, call the prescribing physician or fax the prescribing physician to get authorization to refill.

When refilling prescriptions, be sure it is not too early to refill the medication. If the refill is more than a week early, many insurance companies will refuse to pay and will reject the claim.

Note: Alert the pharmacist if a patient is requesting a refill for a controlled substance too soon.

Refill time is also a good time to check whether a brand name medication can be switched to a generic equivalent.

ACTIVITY

Perform the following:

1. Role-play a telephone call from a patient who is requesting a refill for Plavix, Rx #456921.
2. You have checked the refill screen on the computer and note there are no refills remaining.
3. Fill out the *Refill Request* form along with the fax cover sheet.
4. Fax this information to the prescribing physician.
5. After refills have been authorized by the physician, add the number of refills to the patient's medication file on the computer.
6. Notify the customer that the prescription is ready and refills were added.

Use the following scenarios to complete the exercises.

Patient: Catelynn Walker

Late Friday afternoon Catelynn Walker (DOB 01/15/1979) called in to GetWell Pharmacy to ask for a refill on her birth control pills. Ms. Walker has no refills left on her prescription for Ortho-Cyclen #28, sig: 1 q d. The last time Catelynn refilled the prescription was on 7/01/06. The original prescription is dated 5/1/06 and was prescribed by Dr. Mark Paulsen.

Doctor's fax number is (402) 111-2222.

1. Because there are no refills available to Ms. Walker, what should you tell her after she requests the refill?
2. Complete the fax refill request for the patient Catelynn Walker.

Patient Jeffery Williams

On Tuesday morning Jeffery Williams (DOB 08/01/1965) called in to GetWell Pharmacy to order a refill for Allegra-D. During the phone call, Mr. Williams explained that he does not take this drug regularly, but because of springtime allergies, he needs a refill! He has not had this prescription refilled since September 15, 2005, and now the prescription is expired. The prescription was prescribed by Dr. Jane Coons.

Doctor's fax number is (402) 222-3332.

3. With a partner, role-play making a phone call to Dr. Jane Coons's office. Ask the office nurse or the office receptionist for a refill of Jeffery Williams's Allegra-D. (Each lab partner should take turns portraying the doctor's office and the pharmacy technician requesting the refill.)
4. What should you tell Mr. Williams regarding the time his prescription will be ready for pickup?
5. Complete the fax refill request for the patient Jeffery Williams.

Patient Patrick Grant

On Saturday afternoon Patrick Grant (DOB 06/07/1932) stopped in at GetWell Pharmacy to pick up a refill for his Nitrostat SL pills. Mr. Grant did not call ahead for the refill because he has always had quick service picking up his prescription as a walk-in customer.

Mr. Grant hands the pharmacy technician his empty pill vial with the label information intact.

The vial label indicates last filled 10/15/2006 by Dr. Bill Smith.

Doctor's fax number is (402) 666-3322.

6. With a partner, role-play calling the doctor's office to request a refill for Patrick Grant's Nitrostat. It is Saturday afternoon, so the office is closed. Leave your request on an answering machine or voice mail.
7. It is essential that Mr. Grant have his Nitrostat pills. Yet, there are no refills indicated on the prescription and the physician's office is closed. What should you tell Mr. Grant? What should the pharmacy manager do to ensure that Mr. Grant has his medication?
8. Complete the fax refill request for the patient Patrick Grant.

QUESTIONS FOR REVIEW

1. If a patient wants additional medication for a C-II prescription, how could this request be granted?

2. What are some tips for calling a refill request into a doctor's office?

3. What are three procedures a pharmacy may use to request a prescription refill for a patient?
   a.
   b.
   c.

GETWELL PHARMACY REFILL REQUEST

Fax Refill Request Sheet: Transfer of HIPAA Sensitive Information

118 Feel Better St.

Omaha, NE

402/779-1881

402/779-1882 (Fax)

Confidentiality Notice: The information contained in this facsimile message and the pages that follow is intended for the exclusive use of the addressee(s) and may contain confidential or privileged information. If you are not the intended recipient, please immediately notify GetWell Pharmacy at the location above and destroy all copies and pages of this facsimile.

Name: _____   **DOB:** _____

Medication: _____   **Quantity:** _____

Sig: _____

Last Refill Date: _____   **Doctor:** _____

Physician Office Reply

Please Refill _____ (date) with _____ additional refills.

Authorizing Physician/Agent Signature _____

GETWELL PHARMACY REFILL REQUEST—CONT'D

GetWell Pharmacy

118 Feel Better St.

Omaha, NE 68137

Phone: 402/779-1881

Fax: 402/779-1882

FAX

To: _____

Fax: _____ **Pages:** _____including this cover sheet

Phone: _____ **Date:** _____

Re: _____

• Urgent
• For Review
• Please Comment
• Please Reply

Confidentiality Notice: The information contained in this facsimile message and the pages that follow is intended for the exclusive use of the addressee(s) and may contain confidential or privileged information. If you are not the intended recipient, please immediately notify GetWell Pharmacy at the location above and destroy all copies and pages of this facsimile.

Student Name _____ Date _____

Lab Partner _____

Grade/Comments _____

_____

Student Comments _____

_____

Refill Data Entry

OBJECTIVES

- Perform the necessary computer functions to enter a prescription refill into a pharmacy software system.

- Demonstrate the ability to comprehend patient information shown by using a pharmacy software system.

Pre-Lab Information

Pharmacy managers want to hire technicians who will make their business more successful. The most desirable pharmacy technicians have specific skills necessary to be successful in the pharmacy arena. Therefore, clearly convey your data entry skills relating to pharmacy-specific software when preparing your resume and when interviewing for prospective career placement. The pharmacy-specific software used in this lab is *Visual SuperScript*. Software is not included with this manual.

DATA ENTRY: REFILLING A RETAIL PRESCRIPTION

1. Place the *Visual SuperScript* CD into your computer.
2. Enter your password and select *Fill Rx's* on the menu screen.
3. Click on the *arrow* next to the *Refill Rx's* icon on the left of the screen/form. This will expand or collapse the submenu.
4. Click on the *Refill by Rx #* tab.

5. In the *Rx no. textbox,* type in the prescription refill number: *201268.*
6. The refill dialog box appears on the screen. Click on the *Refill Auth Request Form* tab. This will automatically generate and print a refill authorization form for Joseph Price's Vasotec. The refill authorization form then may be faxed to the patient's physician, Dr. Lamb.
7. Click on *Copy to New Rx* because this prescription has expired. A new prescription will be created. This new prescription and subsequent refills will need to be authorized by the physician. (The refill authorization form in step 6 is used to authorize refills.)
8. The new prescription number and other prescription information is added automatically to the form/screen.
9. A series of dialog boxes will appear, alerting you to price increases and/or HIPAA. Navigate through these dialog boxes by clicking on *o.k.* or *close.*
10. Highlight the text in the *RPh text box* by using your mouse. Change the RPh (registered pharmacist) initials to your first initial then TECH. For example, Jennifer would be JTECH. Change the prescription date, if needed.
11. Press the *tab* key until you reach the *Available Drug Choices* field. *Double-click* on Vasotec 10 mg tablet.
12. Joseph Price will have "0" *refills ordered.* Continue to press the *tab* key through the remaining fields.
13. You now are prompted to save the prescription information. (Unless otherwise directed by your instructor, choose *Abort* instead of saving the information.)
14. Follow the steps to refill a medication for Brian Davidson and Wilma Flintsone. Hint: Use the *Cus History/Refill tab* (customer history and refill) on the left of the fill screen to look up patient names.
15. Click in the small box under the *R* on the patient refill screen. This allows for selection of medication to be refilled.
16. Answer the following questions.

QUESTIONS FOR REVIEW

1. How does the prescription program prompt you to choose a generic equivalent?

2. What is the sig on Joseph Price's prescription?

3. What company manufacturers the medication refilled in Joseph Price's prescription?

4. What is the price and the co-payment on the Vasotec prescription for Joseph Price?

5. What is the new prescription number that was created for Joseph Price's prescription?

Student Name _____ Date _____

Lab Partner _____

Grade/Comments _____

_____

Student Comments _____

_____

Home Medical Equipment

OBJECTIVES

- Explain the process for submitting an insurance claim for home medical equipment.

- Define home medical equipment, and give appropriate examples.

- Demonstrate helping patients with home medical needs, such as compression stockings and mobility equipment.

Pre-Lab Experience

Pharmacy technicians may need to secure prior authorization from the patient's insurance carrier before the purchase of home medical equipment. Visit *www.cignahealthcare.com*. Type "prior authorization form" into the search box. View the information needed on Cigna's prior authorization form.

Prior Authorization = PA
Home Medical Equipment = HME
Durable Medical Equipment = DME

HOME MEDICAL EQUIPMENT

HME, also called durable medical equipment, is a strong branch of retail pharmacy. Home medical equipment involves equipment, devices, or supplies that aid in mobility and/or personal daily living skills. Home medical equipment and supplies are useful to persons who are ill or injured.

Generally, Medicare and private insurance companies help pay for the equipment that meets the following requirements:

1. Prescribed or ordered by a doctor
2. Medically necessary
3. Appropriate for use in the home
4. Fills a medical need (more than a convenience)
5. Can be used over and over again (durable); this requirement does not apply to medical supplies

A pharmacy technician should have a good overall knowledge of home medical equipment and supplies.

The Process of Submitting a Claim for Home Medical Equipment

1. The patient will have a prescription from the physician for the needed equipment.
   a. A prescription is mandatory for insurance to pay for the claim.
2. A certificate of medical necessity may need to be completed. This is a form required by Medicare and other private insurance carries that allows the patient to use certain home medical equipment prescribed by a doctor.
3. A prior authorization form also may need to be completed before purchase of the equipment. Typically PAs are needed for equipment with a purchase price exceeding $1000.
4. Generally, HME is not taxed.

Note: Although the patient has a prescription for the HME, a pharmacist does not need to approve or check the purchase as is done with a prescription medication.

Helping Patients with Home Medical Equipment Needs

Mobility equipment, such as canes and walkers, is common HME. Follow the listed steps to fit a lab partner for a cane:

ACTIVITY

Student Directions

1. Patient should stand as straight as possible with head tilted back. (This may be difficult for some patients with pain or limitations.)
2. Allow patient's arms to hang naturally at sides.
3. The handle of the cane should line up with the bottom crease of the patient's wrist.

View the website *www.scootermobility.com*, *www.pridemobility.com*, or *www.medicalsupplygroup.com* for a variety of information on mobility equipment.

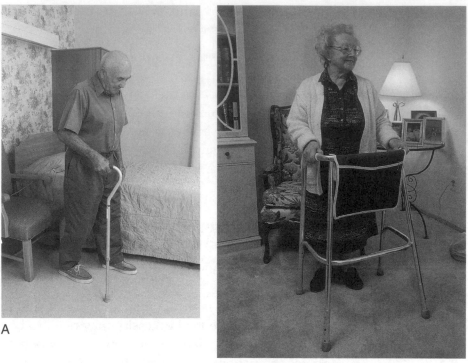

A, Walking with a cane. **B,** Walking with a walker.

ACTIVITY

Another common HME is compression stockings, or support hose used for varicose veins, edema, and postsurgical reasons. A pharmacy technician will be asked to measure the customer for compression stockings.

With a lab partner, follow the guide in correct measuring procedures:

1. The patient should be in a standing position.
2. Using a measuring tape, measure around the smallest part of the ankle. This is the area above the ankle bones.
3. Next, measure around the fullest part of the calf.
4. For knee-high compression stockings measure from the floor to the bend in the back of the knee.
5. For thigh-high compression stockings, measure around the fullest part of the patient's calf.
6. For thigh-high compression stockings, measure from the floor to the top of the thigh.
7. The pharmacy technician will use these measurements to determine the size of stockings needed for the patient, by reading the sizing chart on the compression stocking box.

ACTIVITY

Visit the following website on compression stockings:
http://supporthosestore.com/supwearben.html.

Answer the following questions:

1. Compression stockings are measured in mmHg. What does this mean?

2. At what degree of compression is a prescription needed? Less than 20 mmHg or greater than 20 mmHg?

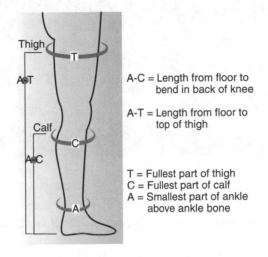

Thigh

T

A•T

Calf

C

A•C

A

A-C = Length from floor to bend in back of knee

A-T = Length from floor to top of thigh

T = Fullest part of thigh
C = Fullest part of calf
A = Smallest part of ankle above ankle bone

3. Visit the following website: *www.independentathome.com.*
4. List products and a feature of the product for each HME category. Bathroom Safety

   Mobility

   Personal Care/Daily Living Aids

5. With a lab partner, role-play the following scenarios:
   A customer asks for your help in finding postsurgical "nylons." The customer seems to be a little confused on exactly what is needed. How would you, as a pharmacy technician, communicate with this customer?

Student Name _____ Date _____

Lab Partner _____

Grade/Comments _____

_____

Student Comments _____

_____

Glucose Monitor

OBJECTIVES

- Demonstrate blood glucose testing procedure.

- Become familiar with blood glucose monitoring supplies.

Pre-Lab Experience

Learn about type 1 and type 2 diabetes.

1. Visit the American Diabetes Association website: *www.diabetes.org*.
2. At the American Diabetes Association home page, click on *For Health Professionals and Scientists*, located on the left side of the page.
3. Click on *Resources for Professionals*.
4. View the five clips: "Diabetes"; "Insulin: The Movie"; "Type One Diabetes"; "Type Two Diabetes"; and "What Happens in Type Two Diabetes?"

BLOOD GLUCOSE MONITORING

The goal of managing diabetes is to maintain normal blood glucose levels. Patients monitor their own blood glucose levels by the use of a blood glucose monitoring machine. These levels then are documented by the patient in a daily logbook.

As a pharmacy technician, it is necessary to be familiar with the monitoring process. Customers will ask for your assistance in purchasing diabetic supplies. Additionally, having knowledge of diabetic monitoring devices will increase your value as a member of the health care team. The staff pharmacist will respect your knowledge in the area of glucose monitoring and will appreciate your assistance with customers/patients.

Blood Testing Procedure

Before performing the following steps, read through the illustrated instruction guide that accompanies the blood glucose monitor kit.

1. Insert a new lancet into the lancet holder cup.
2. Insert a new test strip into the meter.
3. Hold the lancing device on the test site to obtain a blood sample.
4. Apply the blood sample to the test strip.
5. Verify the blood glucose test result by viewing the monitor display screen.

Blood Glucose Range

TIME OF DAY	GLUCOSE RANGE FOR PERSONS WITHOUT DIABETES OR NORMAL LEVEL (mg/dL)	TAKE ACTION (mg/dL)
Preprandial	70-110	<70 and >140
Postprandial	<160	>180
Bedtime	<110	<70 and >160

Application

1. With a lab partner, demonstrate the correct blood testing procedure.
2. Visit the following website to become familiar with blood glucose monitoring devices and supplies: *www.americandiabeteswholesale.com*
3. Read the related document *Blood Glucose Monitoring: Less Pain, More Gain,* by Yvette C. Terrie at *www.pharmacytimes.com/issue/pharmacy/2005/2005-02/2005-02-9282.*
4. Provide answers to the following questions.

QUESTIONS FOR REVIEW

1. How is the daily log blood glucose recording book set up?

2. What is the most important step to achieving control of diabetes?

3. True or false: Advances in lancet devices make it less painful to obtain a blood sample.

4. List three features a patient should look for when selecting a glucose meter.
    a.
    b.
    c.

5. True or false: Reuse lancets when testing to save on health care costs.

6. Where should blood samples be obtained from in order to reduce pain?

7. What should be done to prevent dryness and cracking of skin associated with blood glucose testing?

Student Name _____ Date _____

Lab Partner _____

Grade/Comments _____

_____

Student Comments _____

_____

Automated Dispensing Systems: Baker Cells

OBJECTIVES

- Become familiar with automated dispensing systems used in the pharmacy.

- Identify information needed for Baker Cell documentation.

Pre-Lab Experience

Automated drug dispensing devices (ADDDs) help the pharmacy increase efficiency and enhance patient safety. By using automated dispensing systems such as scales or counting machines, pharmacy personnel save time that then can be spent with the patient. McKesson is a leading provider of automation solutions. Visit their website at *www.mckessonaps.com*. Investigate the automated systems offered by McKesson by clicking on for pharmacies. View the graphics and read descriptions of each system.

Your classroom lab may not be equipped with automated dispensing systems. Therefore, it is important to make note of automated systems when touring pharmacy settings for class.

AUTOMATED DISPENSING SYSTEMS

Baker Cells are compact, automated machines that are used to count pills mechanically. Easy to operate, Baker Cells increase productivity; they count up to 10 capsules or tablets per second. The workflow efficiency of Baker Cassettes helps the pharmacy fill more prescriptions in less time. The system is simple to operate, easily maintained, and extremely durable. Prescriptions are dispensed quickly and accurately with the touch of a button.

Baker Cells or other machines that automatically count pills must be maintained. As a pharmacy technician, you may be in charge of cleaning, stocking, and maintaining the machines.

To clean Baker Cells, use the lint-free wipe and solution provided by the manufacturer. The hopper should be wiped down to remove pill residue. The frequency of cleaning of each Baker Cell depends on the type of medication within the hopper. For instance, Baker Cell hoppers containing hydrocodone are cleaned weekly.

ACTIVITY

1. Fill out two Unit Compliance Records for the Baker Cells. The Unit Compliance Records in this lab are similar to the records you will complete in the pharmacy setting when stocking, maintaining, and cleaning the automated machines.
    a. Cephalexin 250 mg, Cell 1, capsule form, Merck Manufacturer, NDC 12534-1234-01, Quantity: bottle of 100 (five bottles to add), lot number 12345, expiration date: 12/2010.
    b. Allegra 180 mg, Cell 2, tablet form, Watson Pharma Manufacturer, NDC 12345-7894-11, Quantity: bottle of 200 (three bottles to add), lot number 45678, expiration date: 11/2010.

QUESTIONS FOR REVIEW

1. What are two reasons to use automated dispensing machines in an inpatient pharmacy?

2. What are three primary reasons to use automated dispensing machines in an outpatient pharmacy?

3. An automated system used in hospitals that has arms to scan bar codes is called _____.

4. How often should the Baker Cells or another kind of automatic dispensing machine be cleaned?

5. What does NDC stand for?

6. What do the series of numbers in an NDC represent?

7. Explain what the lot number of a medication product means.

Student Name _____ Date _____

Lab Partner _____

Grade/Comments _____

_____

Student Comments _____

_____

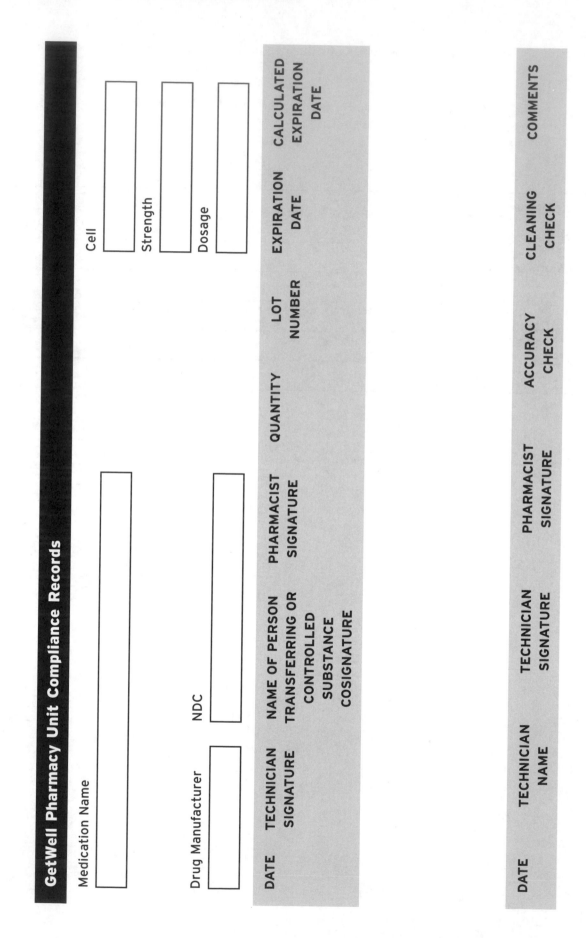

GetWell Pharmacy Unit Compliance Records

Medication Name

Cell

Strength

Drug Manufacturer

NDC

Dosage

DATE	TECHNICIAN SIGNATURE	NAME OF PERSON TRANSFERRING OR CONTROLLED SUBSTANCE COSIGNATURE	PHARMACIST SIGNATURE	QUANTITY	LOT NUMBER	EXPIRATION DATE	CALCULATED EXPIRATION DATE

DATE	TECHNICIAN NAME	TECHNICIAN SIGNATURE	PHARMACIST SIGNATURE	ACCURACY CHECK	CLEANING CHECK	COMMENTS

Health Insurance Portability and Accountability Act (HIPAA)

OBJECTIVES

- Explain the background of HIPAA as it relates to the pharmacy setting.

- Identify HIPAA standards through role-playing exercises.

Pre-Lab Experience

A paper HIPAA notice must be given to pharmacy customers. The HIPAA notice tells the customer how the pharmacy uses and shares his or her health information. The customer should receive the HIPAA notice on his or her first visit to the pharmacy.

Assignment: Acquire at least two HIPAA notices from local pharmacies. Use these HIPAA notices to help with lab exercises.

HEALTH INSURANCE PORTABILITY AND ACCOUNTABILITY ACT

The Health Insurance Portability and Accountability Act (HIPAA) of 1996 established national standards to protect the privacy of personal health care information. HIPAA standards became effective in 2001 with implementation to begin in 2003. As a pharmacy technician, it is your responsibility to keep patient information confidential.

ACTIVITY

Student Directions

Review the attached HIPAA information and the HIPAA notices that were acquired in the pre-lab experience. Answer the following questions by *highlighting* the answer content in your HIPAA information. The answer to question one has been highlighted for you.

1. If a patient asks for a list of medication history, is the pharmacy responsible for supplying the list to the patient? How long does the pharmacy have to furnish the customer with the list?
2. What are the consumers' rights regarding their health information?
3. Highlight topics that are found under the uses and disclosures in your HIPAA notice pamphlet.
4. When is the information in the pamphlet effective?

With your lab partner role-play the following scenario:

A new customer comes into GetWell Pharmacy. Offer the GetWell Pharmacy HIPAA brochure/pamphlet to the new customer, explaining why the customer is getting the HIPAA information. Briefly explain the customer's rights as outlined in HIPAA standards.

HIPAA NOTICE

Providers and health insurers who are required to follow this law must comply with your right to . . . Privacy is important to all of us.

You have privacy rights under a federal law that protects your health information. These rights are important for you to know. You can exercise these rights, ask questions about them, and file a complaint if you think your rights are being denied or your health information is not being protected.

Who must follow this law?
- Most doctors, nurses, pharmacies, hospitals, clinics, nursing homes, and many other health care providers
- Health insurance companies, HMOs, and most employer group health plans
- Certain government programs that pay for health care, such as Medicare and Medicaid

Ask to see and get a copy of your health records
You can ask to see and get a copy of your medical record and other health information. You may not be able to get all of your information in a few special cases. For example, if your doctor decides something in your file might endanger you or someone else, the doctor may not have to give this information to you.
- In most cases, your copies must be given to you within 30 days, but this can be extended for another 30 days if you are given a reason.
- You may have to pay for the cost of copying and mailing if you request copies and mailing.

Have corrections added to your health information
You can ask to change any wrong information in your file or add information to your file if it is incomplete. For example, if you and your hospital agree that your file has the wrong result for a test, the hospital must change it. Even if the hospital believes the test result is correct, you still have the right to have your disagreement noted in your file.

- In most cases the file should be changed within 60 days, but the hospital can take an extra 30 days if you are given a reason.

Receive a notice that tells you how your health information is used and shared
You can learn how your health information is used and shared by your provider or health insurer. They must give you a notice that tells you how they may use and share your health information and how you can exercise your rights. In most cases, you should get this notice on your first visit to a provider or in the mail from your health insurer, and you can ask for a copy at any time.

Decide whether to give your permission before your information can be used or shared for certain purposes
In general, your health information cannot be given to your employer, used or shared for things like sales calls or advertising, or used or shared for many other purposes unless you give your permission by signing an authorization form. This authorization form must tell you who will get your information and what your information will be used for.

Published by the U.S. Department of Health & Human Services Office for Civil Rights.

Other privacy rights

You may have other health information rights under your state's laws. When these laws affect how your health information can be used or shared, that should be made clear in the notice you receive.

For more information
This is a brief summary of your rights and protections under the federal health information privacy law. You can ask your provider or health insurer questions about how your health information is used or shared and about your rights. You also can learn more, including how to file a complaint with the U.S. Government, at the

website at *www.hhs.gov/ocr/hipaa/* or by calling 1-866-627-7748; the phone call is free.

Get a report on when and why your health information was shared

Under the law, your health information may be used and shared for particular reasons, like making sure doctors give good care, making sure nursing homes are clean and safe, reporting when the flu is in your area, or making required reports to the police, such as reporting gunshot wounds. In many cases, you can ask for and get a list of whom your health information has been shared with for these reasons.

- You can get this report for free once a year.
- In most cases you should get the report within 60 days, but it can take an extra 30 days if you are given a reason.

Ask to be reached somewhere other than home

You can make reasonable requests to be contacted at different places or in a different way. For example, you can have the nurse call you at your office instead of your home, or send mail to you in an envelope instead of on a postcard. If sending information to you at home might put you in danger, your health insurer must talk, call, or write to you where you ask and in the way you ask, if the request is reasonable.

Ask that your information not be shared

You can ask your provider or health insurer not to share your health information with certain people, groups, or companies. For example, if you go to a clinic, you could ask the doctor not to share your medical record with other doctors or nurses in the clinic. However, they do not have to agree to do what you ask.

File complaints

If you believe your information was used or shared in a way that is not allowed under the privacy law, or if you were not able to exercise your rights, you can file a complaint with your provider or health insurer. The privacy notice you receive from them will tell you who to talk to and how to file a complaint. You can also file a complaint with the U.S. Government.

The Law Gives You Rights over Your Health Information

Most of us feel that our health and medical information is private and should be protected, and we want to know who has this information. Now, federal law

- Gives you rights over your health information
- Sets rules and limits on who can look at and receive your health information

Who must follow this law?

- Most doctors, nurses, pharmacies, hospitals, clinics, nursing homes, and many other health care providers
- Health insurance companies, HMOs, and most employer group health plans
- Certain government programs that pay for health care, such as Medicare and Medicaid

What information is protected?

- Information your doctors, nurses, and other health care providers put in your medical record
- Conversations your doctor has about your care or treatment with nurses and others
- Information about you in your health insurer's computer system
- Billing information about you at your clinic
- Most other health information about you held by those who must follow this law

Providers and health insurers who are required to follow this law must comply with your right to

- Ask to see and get a copy of your health records
- Have corrections added to your health information
- Receive a notice that tells you how your health information may be used and shared
- Decide if you want to give your permission before your health information can be used or shared for certain purposes, such as for marketing
- Get a report on when and why your health information was shared for certain purposes
- If you believe your rights are being denied or your health information is not being protected, you can

- File a complaint with your provider or health insurer
- File a complaint with the U.S. Government

You should get to know these important rights, which help you protect your health information. You can ask your provider or health insurer questions about your rights. You also can learn more about your rights, including how to file a complaint, from the website at *www.hhs.gov/ocr/hipaa/* or by calling 1-866-627-7748; the phone call is free.

The Law Protects the Privacy of Your Health Information

Providers and health insurers who are required to follow this law must keep your information private by
- Teaching the people who work for them how your information may and may not be used and shared
- Taking appropriate and reasonable steps to keep your health information secure

To make sure that your information is protected in a way that does not interfere with your health care, your information can be used and shared
- For your treatment and care coordination
- To pay doctors and hospitals for your health care and help run their businesses
- With your family, relatives, friends, or others you identify who are involved with your health care or your health care bills, unless you object
- To make sure doctors give good care and nursing homes are clean and safe
- To protect the public's health, such as by reporting when the flu is in your area
- To make required reports to the police, such as reporting gunshot wounds

Your health information cannot be used or shared without your written permission unless this law allows it. For example, without your authorization, your provider generally cannot
- Give your information to your employer
- Use or share your information for marketing or advertising purposes
- Share private notes about your mental health counseling sessions

Published by the U.S. Department of Health & Human Services Office for Civil Rights.

This is a brief summary of your rights and protections under the federal health information privacy law. You can learn more about health information privacy and your rights in a fact sheet called "Your Health Information Privacy Rights." You can get this from the website at *www.hhs.gov/ocr/hipaa/*. You can also call 1-866-627-7748; the phone call is free.

Other privacy rights

Another law provides additional privacy protections to patients of alcohol and drug treatment programs. For more information, go to the website at *www.samhsa.gov.*

Student Name _____ Date _____

Lab Partner _____

Grade/Comments _____

_____

Student Comments _____

_____

Mail Order

OBJECTIVE

- Distinguish prescription filling process in a mail-order pharmacy from other pharmacy settings.

Pre-Lab Information

A pharmacy technician has the benefit of a variety of settings in which to work. What working conditions can a pharmacy technician expect in a mail-order pharmacy? Typically, the work environment takes a relaxed tone. The dress code will be casual attire. You can expect traditional working hours of Monday through Friday, 8 AM to 6 PM, with an occasional Saturday work day. Some mail-order pharmacies may provide service to a few walk-in customers. Otherwise, plan on little contact with the public in a mail-order pharmacy.

MAIL-ORDER PRESCRIPTIONS

The prescription filling process in a mail-order pharmacy is as follows:

Mail Room
- The majority of prescription orders are received in a mail-order pharmacy. A small number are received by phone, fax, or Internet.

Data Entry
- Patient and insurance information is entered into the computer.
    - Patient information includes safety cap preference, brand or generic preference, allergy and disease information, and shipping preference.

Order Entry
- Prescription data are entered into the computer.

Filling or Dispensing
- Prescription orders are filled.

Checking Area
- Finished prescriptions are checked by the pharmacist.

Shipping Area
- When mailing prescriptions out to customers, the pharmacy technician will be responsible for completing invoices, mail logs, and charge logs as well as cross-checking the invoice with the prescriptions being mailed. This is done by checking the medication name on the vial with the drug name and quantity listed on the invoice.
- The prescription order then is packaged in a bubble wrap envelope with corresponding literature. The order is mailed in a box if the medication needs to be on ice.

Medications dispensed in nonlock lids are sealed to prevent accidental opening in the mail. This is done by placing tape over the lid.

QUESTIONS FOR REVIEW

1. Review the steps for mailing medications.
    a.
    b.
    c.
    d.
    e.
    f.
    g.
    h.

2. Why is it necessary to take the time to document mail-order medications?

3. Provide examples of clientele who would use mail order.

ACTIVITY

4. Using the two mail-order scenarios, role-play with a lab partner. Prepare the written documentation that is needed for medications to be mailed out for the following patients.
   a. Invoice
   b. Mail log
   c. First-party charge log
   d. Address mailing envelope (envelope provided by your instructor)

Scenario 1

Patient Chris Karver calls into Getwell Pharmacy on Monday, January 5, 2007. Mr. Karver desires a refill for his medication, giving the pharmacy technician the prescription number 68756. Mr. Karver asks the pharmacy technician to mail the prescription along with a bottle of baby aspirin. Chris Karver's address is 12214 Dodge Street, Omaha, NE 68154.

Scenario 2

A prescription order is received via facsimile for Megan Plusa.

Dr. Mark Paulsen   office: 800/777-2211
2100 Lake Avenue
Farmview, IA 51223

  Patient Name__Megan Plusa_____   **Date**__5/7/07_____
  Address___1391 Orchard Lane   Fremont, MO_____

                                          Refill___7____Times

      Rx: Glucophage 500mg TID
         #90

Dr. Mark Paulsen

Product Selection Permitted   **Dispense As Written**

DEA NO._____
Address_____

INVOICE NUMBER

100__

GetWell Pharmacy Invoice
11818 I Street
Omaha, NE 68137

Name of Customer
Address
City, State

Total Due: $_____

Description of Charges
*List Rx Number Only to
Protect the Privacy of the
Patient (HIPAA)*

Quantity

Price

SUBTOTAL _____
TAX (7%) _____
(No Tax on Rx) _____
TOTAL _____

GetWell Pharmacy Charge Log					
INVOICE NUMBER	DATE	CUSTOMER NAME	AMOUNT CHARGED	DATE PAID	LOGGER'S INITIALS

GetWell Pharmacy Mail Log

DATE	AM PM	CUSTOMER NAME	CUSTOMER ADDRESS	RX#	INVOICE #	OWE/SHORTAGE	PHARMACY TECH INITIALS

Student Name _____ Date _____

Lab Partner _____

Grade/Comments _____

_____

Student Comments _____

_____

Inpatient Pharmacy

Processing Inpatient Prescriptions

OBJECTIVE

- Evaluate information needed on inpatient/acute care medication orders.

Pre-Lab Experience

On prescription orders in the acute care setting, it is essential to include the patient's date of birth (DOB) and the patient's weight. The safe practice of including these two pieces of patient information on prescription orders will ensure correct milligram per kilogram (mg/kg) dosing. The safe practice of including DOB on drug orders ensures correct pediatric dosing and geriatric considerations.

1. Visit the website for the Institute for Safe Medication Practices at *www.ismp.org/newsletters/acutecare/articles/default.asp*.
2. Perform a search titled *hospital medication orders*.
3. Read the article *ISMP: Medication Safety Alert!*
4. List three error prevention strategies as stated in the article *ISMP: Medication Safety Alert!*
   a.
   b.
   c.

INPATIENT PRESCRIPTIONS: MEDICATION ORDER

In the hospital or inpatient pharmacy the medication order is the equivalent of the prescription in the retail pharmacy. When a patient is hospitalized, all prescription and over-the-counter medications require a medication order from the physician.

An appropriately written medication order must include the following information:

- Patient's name, height, and weight
- Patient's hospital room number and identification number
- Diagnosis
- Known allergies
- Medication name, strength, dosage form, route, and directions
- Attending physician's name and signature

ACTIVITY

Student Directions

Using a highlighter marker, indicate information that is missing or incomplete from each inpatient order.

Patient: Newman, Patricia DOB: 1-09-60 Sex: F Chart NO: Allergies: NKA Diagnosis: Physician: Dr. Mark Paulsen	**MEMORIAL HOSPITAL** Exira, Iowa **Physician Order Record**

	10/10/06 0800
	Admit to acute care:
	Diet: DAT
	Activity: ad lib
	Meds: Coumadin 2 mg q am, MVI q am, Demerol 50 mg PO q 3-4 h prn pain
	Labs: CBC in am
	Dr. Paulsen

Patient: Sander, Rebecca **Room #:** 109B **DOB:** 03-09-1958 **Sex:** F **Chart NO:** **Allergies:** Morphine **Diagnosis:** ABD Pain **Physician:** Dr. Megan Wickland	**MEMORIAL HOSPITAL** Exira, Iowa **Physician Order Record**

6/3/06 1300

Admit to OP

Activity: BR

Diet: Diabetic ADA

ABD US on admit

Meds: Metformin 500 mg PO tid

ASA 81 mg qd

Tyl 500 mg PO q4h prn pain

NPO for now   *Dr. John Thompson*

Nursing to obtain pt ht and wt

Ht: 5'4"

Wt: 116 lb

ACTIVITY

Using the inpatient medication order for Rebecca Sander, perform the steps listed for filling an inpatient order:

1. A copy of the original medication order is received in the pharmacy.
2. The pharmacy technician must distinguish between medication and nonmedication orders.
3. Medication orders are transcribed and are entered into the computer system.
4. The pharmacy technician compares and checks the original medication order with the computer-generated label.
5. The label then is taken to the shelf to locate the correct unit dose medication.
6. The correct single, unit dose medication is selected for the individual patient.
7. A 24-hour supply of unit dose medication is prepared for the individual patient.
8. Unit dose medication is placed inside a plastic bag that has been labeled with the patient's name, identification number, and room number.
9. Notify the pharmacist that the patient medication is ready to be checked.
10. Patient medication is replenished in the nursing unit medicine cart on a scheduled basis. Stat medication orders and patient medication that is needed before the scheduled medicine cart fill will be delivered to the patient care unit according to hospital protocol.

Student Name _____ Date _____

Lab Partner _____

Grade/Comments _____

_____

Student Comments _____

_____

Automation

OBJECTIVE

• Discover the benefits of pharmacy automation.

Pre-Lab Experience

Pharmacy technicians and other pharmacy personnel have the challenge of maintaining the highest standards in patient safety. Pharmacy personnel must focus on meeting customer needs. At the same time, quality health care should not be jeopardized. Two goals of pharmacy technology are to enhance efficiency and ensure patient safety. Learn about pharmacy technology by logging onto *www.mckesson.com*

How does McKesson handle medication management in the hospital setting?

How does McKesson partner with retail pharmacy to enhance accuracy?

PHARMACY TECHNOLOGY

In any pharmacy setting, automation is part of the pharmacy technician's daily schedule. The evolution of automation and robotics in the pharmacy provides many benefits. Most important is the positive trend toward reduction of medication errors.

ACTIVITY

1. Using the Internet, access *www.Rxinsider.com*
2. Scroll down the home page, and investigate the following:
   a. Dispensing Systems
   b. Automated Prescription Systems
   c. Tablet/Capsule Counters
   d. Bar Coding
   e. Unit Dose Packaging
   f. Label Printing Software
   g. Medication Carts
   h. Robotic Systems
   i. Thermal Medication Packaging and Sealing
3. Write a short paragraph describing what you learned about each of these systems.

Student Name _____ Date _____

Lab Partner _____

Grade/Comments _____

_____

Student Comments _____

_____

Extemporaneous Compounding

LAB

17

Part I: Balance

OBJECTIVE

- Demonstrate use of a Class A prescription balance.

Pre-Lab Experience

Visit http://apothecaryproducts.dirxion.com and use the search field to see various models of pharmacy balances such as the torsion balance and the electronic balance. List three accessory items that are needed when working with a prescription balance.

1.

2.

3.

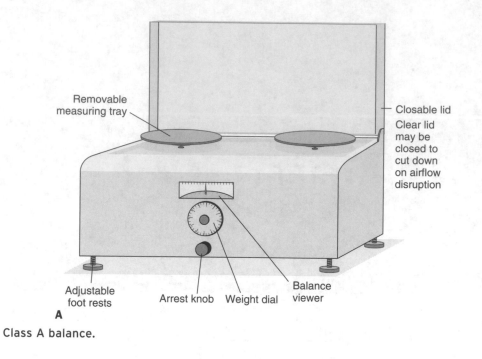

Class A balance.

EXTEMPORANEOUS COMPOUNDING: PART I

Class A Prescription Balance

A balance is used to determine the weight of a dosage form. The Class A balance is a two-pan torsion-type balance. The set of metric weights must always be handled with forceps and stored in its box. To obtain an accurate weight of dosage form, appropriate techniques must be used.

1. Lock the balance by turning the arrest knob.
2. The black dial located on the front of the balance should be at zero. This dial is used if a weight set does not have small-increment weights. For example; if the compounding order calls for 1.2 g, place a 1-g weight on the pan and set the dial to 0.2 for a total weight of 1.2 g. Always use the balance on a level surface.
3. Level the balance front to back by turning the leveling screw feet until the leveling bubble is in the middle of the tube.
4. Turn the calibrated dial to zero.
5. Unlock the balance and adjust the screw feet if needed until the pointer rests at the center of the marker plate.
6. Lock the balance. Then place weighing paper on each pan.
7. Unlock the balance by releasing the arrest knob. If needed, level the balance.
8. Lock the balance, and place the required weights on the weighing paper on the right pan.
9. Using a spatula, place the material to be weighed on the weighing paper in the left pan.

10. Unlock the balance. If the pointer has shifted to the left or right, adjust the dosage material.
11. Always arrest the balance before adding or removing weight from either pan.

1. Practice using a Class A prescription balance and a mortar and pestle. Prepare the following amounts of ingredients:

   a. 2.75 g ground cinnamon
   b. 8.5 g sugar
   c. 2.5 g triturated clove

2. Combine the ingredients, and use the punch method to fill capsules with this compound.

Student Name _____ Date _____

Lab Partner _____

Grade/Comments _____

_____

Student Comments _____

_____

Part II: Compounding

OBJECTIVE

- Become familiar with basic compounding equipment.

Pre-Lab Experience

Take a quick look back in history at pharmacy compounding equipment used in 1920 through 1950. Visit Sea View Hospital Healthcare Museum at *www.seaviewmuseum.org*. Click on *pharmacy*. Click on the thumbnail images to view compounding items.

EXTEMPORANEOUS COMPOUNDING: PART II

Compounding has various aspects. Compounding can mean the preparation of suspensions, the conversion of one dosage form into another, preparing pediatric dosage forms from adult dosage forms, intravenous admixtures, and suppositories. Extemporaneous compounding is the on-demand preparation of a drug product according to a given formula or recipe.

1. Become familiar with basic compounding equipment in the retail lab area.
   a. Spatula
   b. Mortar
   c. Pestle
   d. Graduated cylinder

    e. Parchment paper
    f. Weighing papers or boats
    g. Class A balance
2. Practice your compounding technique.
    a. Measure liquid
        i. In the graduated cylinder: 15 mL, 50 mL, 250 mL
        ii. In the amber oval or bottle: 4 oz, 160 mL
    b. Unit dose
        i. Using OPUS cassettes
        ii. Using the bubble pack
    c. Punch method with capsules
        i. Place 2 g corn starch in capsule
    d. Reconstitute
3. Reinforce your understanding of information needed on a compounded product label by correctly labeling material that has been compounded.
4. Practice extemporaneous documentation by completing the pharmacy log sheet that is labeled *Master Formula Sheet*.
5. Answer questions for review.

QUESTIONS FOR REVIEW

1. Why is it important to compound only one product at a time?
    a. To reduce chance of error
    b. To increase speed in compounding
    c. To make better use of inventory
2. An example of a patient who may have medication prepared unit dose is _____.
    a. An elderly patient in a nursing home
    b. A patient who wishes to save money
    c. A patient who is unable to open pill bottles
3. What dosage form may you be asked to compound for a young child?
    a. Tablet
    b. Oral syrup
    c. Capsule
4. What auxiliary label is needed for a suspension that should be stored at 2° to 8° C?
    a. Do not shake.
    b. Shake well.
    c. Keep refrigerated.

MASTER FORMULA SHEET

Manufactured Product Information:

Name of Preparation _____

Product Assigned Lot Number _____

Date Product Manufactured _____

Expiration Dating _____

Quantity Manufactured _____

Strength/Dosage Form _____

Storage Instructions:

Label for Product (Include any auxiliary label that may be needed):

Manufacturer's Lot Number	Ingredient and Strength	Amount Needed	Weighed or Measured by	Checked by

Directions for Manufacturing (may use recipe for product as a guide):

Product Manufactured/Prepared by: _____

Approving Pharmacist _____

Student Name _____ Date _____

Lab Partner _____

Grade/Comments _____

_____

Student Comments _____

_____

Part III: Compounding

OBJECTIVE

- Become capable of performing extemporaneous compounding technique.

Pre-Lab Experience

Find out more about extemporaneous compounding by visiting the Professional Compounding Centers of America (PCCA) website: *www.pccarx.com.*

Click on *Resources for Pharmacists.*

How has pharmacy compounding changed through the years?

According to the PCCA, what is the most important reason for compounding prescription medications?

EXTEMPORANEOUS COMPOUNDING: PART III

Name of preparation: Spicy Ointment
Strength/quantity of preparation: 30 g
Dosage form: Ointment
Ingredients:

    Spice   1 g
    Cetaphil   29 g

Expiration dating: 6-month version
Storage instructions:
Store at room temperature.
Compounding instructions:
Gather the following items:

    Parchment paper
    Spatula
    Cetaphil
    Spice
    Empty 1-oz ointment jar

Fill out the compounding record or Master Formula Sheet.

Lay out the sheet of parchment paper on a flat surface. It may be easier to mix the components if the edges of the paper are taped to the counter, so that it will not move while mixing.

Using the spatula, scrape out the desired amount of Cetaphil from the ointment jar, and place it on one side of the parchment paper.

With the spatula, separate out a small amount of the Cetaphil to form a small pile. Then, add weighed spice onto the separated Cetaphil.

Use the flat, metal side of the spatula blade to mix the two components together. Push down on the handle of the spatula and smooth the ointment from side to side. If performed correctly, the metal of the spatula will bow slightly because of the pressure as you push down and side to side to mix the ointment.

When mixed, add more of the Cetaphil and additional amounts of spice into what you have already mixed. Mix well with the spatula.

Continue to add the two components, little by little, until both ingredients are mixed completely. This technique is called *geometric dilution.*

Once both ingredients have been incorporated thoroughly, carefully scoop the ointment into the appropriately labeled, empty ointment jar using the spatula. Avoid getting ointment on the outside of the jar. Screw the cap on tightly.

MASTER FORMULA SHEET

Manufactured Product Information:

Name of Preparation_____

Product Assigned Lot Number_____

Date Product Manufactured_____

Expiration Dating_____

Quantity Manufactured_____

Strength/Dosage Form_____

Storage Instructions:

Label for Product (Include any auxiliary label that may be needed):

Manufacturer's Lot Number	Ingredient and Strength	Amount Needed	Weighed or Measured By	Checked By

Directions for Manufacturing: (May use recipe for product as a guide).

Product Manufactured/Prepared by: _____

Approving Pharmacist _____

QUESTIONS FOR REVIEW

1. Which of the following pieces of equipment is used to compound Spicy Ointment?
   a. Spatula
   b. Mortar and pestle
   c. Counting tray
   d. 4-oz oval

2. Which describes the mixing of both components of this ointment?
   a. Levigation
   b. Trituration
   c. Geometric dilution
   d. Repackaging
3. The spice should be added _____.
   a. One half of the total amount first, then the second half
   b. All at once
   c. Quickly
   d. Small amounts at a time
4. What auxiliary label should be applied to the Spicy Ointment dispensing container?
   a. Shake well.
   b. Keep refrigerated.
   c. For topical use only.
   d. Take with food.
5. To ensure stability, Spicy Ointment should be stored at _____.
   a. 30° to 40° C
   b. 15° to 30° C
   c. 2° to 8° C
   d. −20° to −10° C

Student Name _____ Date _____

Lab Partner _____

Grade/Comments _____

_____

Student Comments _____

_____

Part IV: Compounding

OBJECTIVE

- Demonstrate basic knowledge of extemporaneous compounding techniques.

Pre-Lab Experience

Compounded prescriptions are ideal for any patient requiring unique dosages and/or dosage forms such as solutions, suppositories, sprays, oral rinses, or lollipops. Sometimes patients need medicine at strengths that are not manufactured by drug companies. Compounding provides a way to customize prescriptions for the specific need of a patient. Examples of commonly compounded medications are hormone replacement therapy, pediatric dosing, and combining multiple medications into a single, more convenient dose that helps patients with chronic pain management.

Visit Gallipot website at *www.gallipot.com*.

Listed under *Browse Categories*, click on *Bases/Vehicles* Then select *topical*. Scroll through the name and description of products available. Give a brief description of methylcellulose 1%. The *Equipment/Supplies* link on the Gallipot website shows compounding equipment such as balances, beakers, capsule machines, and molds.

SUPPLIES NEEDED

Mortar and pestle
4-oz oval
Master Formula Sheet
Recipe ingredients

EXTEMPORANEOUS COMPOUNDING: PART IV

Name of preparation: Judy's Suspension
Strength/quantity of preparation: 125 mg/5 mL; 120 mL
Dosage form: Oral suspension
Ingredients:

Smarties	#6: 500 mg each
Distilled water	15 mL
O.K. Oil	30 mL
Sweet liquid	qs to 120 mL

Expiration dating: 6-month version
Storage instructions:
Store under refrigeration.
Compounding instructions:
Gather the following items:

Mortar and pestle
Smarties
Sweet liquid
O.K. Oil
Distilled water
Empty 120-mL oval labeled for suspension

Fill out the compounding record or Master Formula Sheet.

Pulverize #6, 500-mg Smarties tablets with mortar and pestle, making certain to grind to a very fine powder. Then add 15 mL of distilled water to mortar and continue gently mixing with pestle. Carefully pour contents of mortar into the appropriately labeled, empty 4-oz. plastic amber oval.

Add 30 mL of suspending agent (O.K. Oil) to oval. Swirl vigorously to mix contents.

QS to 120 mL with Sweet Oil. Shake well.

MASTER FORMULA SHEET

Manufactured Product Information:

Name of Preparation _____

Product Assigned Lot Number _____

Date Product Manufactured _____

Expiration Dating _____

Quantity Manufactured _____

Strength/Dosage Form _____

Storage Instructions:

Label for Product (Include any auxiliary label that may be needed):

Manufacturer's Lot Number	Ingredient and Strength	Amount Needed	Weighed or Measured by	Checked by

Directions for Manufacturing (may use recipe for product as a guide):

Product Manufactured/Prepared by: _____

Approving Pharmacist _____

QUESTIONS FOR REVIEW

1. When made according to recipe, how many ounces of suspension are made?
   a. 1
   b. 3
   c. 4
   d. 10

2. Which of the following is the suspending agent?
    a. Distilled water
    b. O.K. Oil
    c. Sweet liquid
    d. Smarties

3. What is the concentration of the finished suspension?
    a. 250 mg/mL
    b. 50 mg/5 mL
    c. 125 mg/5 mL
    d. 250 mg/5 mL

4. What would the resulting concentration of the suspension be if #12, 500-mg Smarties tablets were used?
    a. 250 mg/5 mL
    b. 50 mg/mL
    c. Both A and B
    d. 500 mg/5 mL

Student Name _____ Date _____

Lab Partner _____

Grade/Comments _____

_____

Student Comments _____

_____

Aseptic Technique and IV Compounding

Introduction to Aseptic IV Compounding Pharmacy

OBJECTIVES

- Identify and become familiar with compounding pharmacy devices, supplies, and equipment.

- Discover facts about the evolution of antibiotics.

Pre-Lab Experience

1. Take a photo tour of pharmacies of the past by visiting the University of Arizona College of Pharmacy: *www.pharmacy.arizona.edu/visitors/ pharmacy-museum/history-pharmacy-museum-photo-tour*.
2. Learn about the development of chemotherapy drugs, the era of antibiotics, the era of biologicals, and more by touring the Parke, Davis, and Company A History of Pharmacy in Pictures website: *www.pharmacy.wsu.edu/history*.

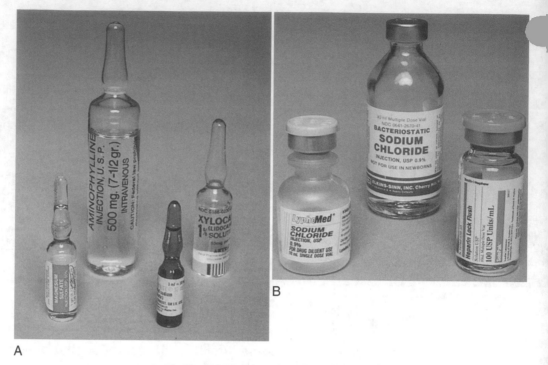

A, Medication in ampules. **B,** Medication in vials.

ORIENTATION TO THE ASEPTIC IV COMPOUNDING LAB

1. Locate the following items in the compounding lab:
   a. Laminar horizontal airflow hood/laminar airflow workbench
   b. Laminar vertical airflow hood/biological safety cabinet
   c. Vials
      i. Multidose and single-dose vials
   d. Ampules
   e. Syringes
      i. Luer-Lok
      ii. Slip-Lok
   f. Needles
   g. Personal protective equipment
   h. Garb
   i. Automated compounding system
   j. Small-volume parenteral bags and large-volume parenteral bags
      i. Ready-to-mix systems

2. List one injectable medication that is contained in any one of the pharmacy compounding lab ampules or vials.

3. What is the needle size, gauge, and length of any one of the needles located in the pharmacy compounding lab?

4. How is the stock medication supply arranged?

5. What syringe volume ranges are available in the pharmacy compounding lab?

Student Name _____ Date _____

Lab Partner _____

Grade/Comments _____

_____

Student Comments _____

_____

Part I: Aseptic Technique

OBJECTIVES

• Become capable of using aseptic technique procedures.

• Demonstrate aseptic hand hygiene technique.

Pre-Lab Experience

CSP: compounded sterile preparations
USP Chapter 797: *United States Pharmacopeia* Chapter 797
ISO: International Standards Organization
Clean room: a room in which the concentration of airborne particles is controlled and that is constructed and used in a manner to minimize the introduction, generation, and retention of particulates inside the room, and in which other relevant parameters—for example, temperature, humidity, and pressure—are controlled as necessary
Airborne contamination: materials in the environment that can affect the health of an individual. The contaminated material consists of small particle residue that may remain suspended in the air for long periods. A contaminated particle may be dispersed by air currents and then become deposited on compounding supplies.

Learn more about clean rooms by visiting the United States Pharmacopeia website: *www.usp.org*.

ASEPTIC TECHNIQUE

Aseptic technique refers to the procedure carried out during the preparation of a sterile product in order to minimize the chance of contamination. Aseptic technique is a technical function for which practice is necessary in order to begin to master the skills needed.

Aseptic technique requires controlling the environment in which compounding is prepared. Horizontal and vertical flow hoods are used to reduce the risk of airborne contamination during compounding preparations.

Working in a horizontal or vertical flow hood does not guarantee a sterile product. The technique to which the pharmacy technician adheres is what helps ensure a safe, sterile end product.

USP Chapter 797 was released in January 2004. With the addition of Chapter 797, a new national standard for sterile preparation was created. The new standards were designed to improve the quality of sterile preparations, which in turn will improve patient safety and reduce the number of adverse events related to compounding practices.

Aseptic technique involves many factors over which the pharmacy technician has control: hand washing, cleaning the laminar flow hood/biological safety cabinet, "gowning up," and placement and handling of materials used during compounding of preparations.

HAND WASHING

1. Review Lab 2, Hand Washing.
2. When working with sterile products, *additional steps* in the hand-washing procedure are necessary.
3. First, remove hand and wrist jewelry.
4. Microbes flourish beneath fingernails; therefore, it is important to keep nails trimmed. Equally important is the added step of scrubbing fingernails.
5. Finally, use appropriate cleanser, and scrub hands and arms to the elbows.
6. Let water drip from the hands to the elbows by holding hands up.

Aseptic Hand-Washing Technique

	YES	NO
Removed all hand and wrist jewelry or other objects from the elbow down		
Did not wear acrylic nails or use nail polish		
Turned on the water and adjusted temperature to the proper level		
Wetted the hands thoroughly with water before applying soap		
Applied the appropriate amount of the proper disinfectant/cleanser		
Thoroughly washed palms, back of hands, fingers, under the fingernails, and wrists for at least 15 seconds		
Rinsed each hand thoroughly, being sure all soap residue was gone		
Held rinsed hands upright so that water dripped to the elbows		
Used a circular motion while drying each hand thoroughly with a dry, clean, lint-free paper towel Used a separate towel or dry portion of the towel for each hand		
Used a clean, dry towel to turn off the faucet handle and clean the sink area		
Did not touch the faucet or sink area directly after washing hands		

Student Name _____ Date _____

Lab Partner _____

Grade/Comments _____

_____

Student Comments _____

_____

Part II: Aseptic Technique

OBJECTIVES

- Become capable of performing aseptic gowning procedure.

- Gain an understanding of the purpose of cleanroom garb.

Pre-Lab Information

Garb: coat or gown, mask, gloves, and shoe covers worn during aseptic compounding

Anteroom: an area adjacent to the cleanroom. The anteroom contains supplies and medication products to be compounded.

ASEPTIC TECHNIQUE: GOWNING

The purpose of cleanroom garb is to keep naturally produced human body particles from contaminating the compounding area. The second and equally important purpose of cleanroom garb is, in some instances, to protect the pharmacy technician from contamination. Aseptic compounding garb consists of a gown or coat with elastic cuffs, hair cover, mask, gloves, and shoe covers. Additional garb is required for higher-risk compounding such as chemotherapy.

Coats: Lab coats worn elsewhere in the pharmacy are not acceptable for compounding areas.

Shoe covers: Shoe covers should be put on before the feet touch the floor on the clean side of the room.

Masks: Masks are put on just before beginning work at the laminar workbench. Masks should be changed each time you reenter the compounding area.

Gloves: Gloves may be latex or vinyl. Avoid powdered gloves because the powder residue can be deposited on supplies. Nitrile gloves may be chosen over vinyl or latex. Nitrile gloves are manufactured using synthetic latex and are 3 times more puncture resistant than natural rubber. They offer superior resistance to punctures and also are used for protection against a variety of chemicals. Nitrile gloves are easy to don (put on) because of the materials of which the gloves are made.

During sterile compounding, thoroughly rinse gloves with a disinfectant such as 70% isopropyl alcohol. Change gloves if punctured, torn, or contaminated. During extended compounding, resanitize your gloves with 70% isopropyl alcohol.

Gowning takes place in the anteroom. Gowning should be performed from the head down. Begin with hair cover; then mask, shoe cover, gown; and then gloves should be put on last. Other than shoe covers, garb should never touch or drag on the floor. Garb should fit properly.

ASEPTIC TECHNIQUE: DE-GOWNING

When leaving a cleanroom, you should discard all of your garb, and on reentry you will use fresh garb. If the pharmacy procedures allow for certain garb to be used again on reentry, these garments should be removed so that the outside of the garment is contaminated as little as possible. Deglove by pulling the glove off, inside out. Use the fingers from the hand that has just been removed from the glove to pull the remaining glove down and over the first removed glove. The shoe covers should be removed one at a time. Then remove the gown or coat by untying and placing hands inside the gown to remove it. Do not let the gown touch the floor. Next, remove the face mask and then the hair cover.

IT IS YOUR RESPONSIBILITY AS A PHARMACY TECHNICIAN TO FOLLOW PROPER GOWNING AND DE-GOWNING PROCEDURES!

Proper Gowning Technique

	YES	NO
Select proper size and type of gown		
Removed all hand and wrist jewelry or other objects from the elbow down		
Properly apply face mask, hair covering, and shoe covers (if necessary)		
Put gown on properly		
Wash hands using aseptic technique		
Put on gloves properly		
De-gowned properly		

Visit *www.coastwidelabs.com*, select *Technical Information/Articles*, and click on "Cleaning the Cleanroom – Contamination Control."

List four "do not" cleanroom guidelines.

1.
2.
3.
4.

Student Name _____ Date _____

Lab Partner _____

Grade/Comments _____

_____

Student Comments _____

_____

Cleaning a Horizontal Laminar Airflow Hood

OBJECTIVES

- Demonstrate the correct technique used to clean a horizontal laminar airflow hood.

- Understand the role of a HEPA filter.

Pre-Lab Information

HEPA: high-efficiency particulate air (filter)
Prefilter: replaceable filters installed before a final filter to remove gross contamination and protect the final filter from environmental conditions. The prefilters have a lower efficiency than the one they protect.
Particulate: pertaining to a minute particle or fragment of a substance or material

1. Learn more about HEPA filters by visiting the website *www.hepafilters.com*.

Click on *Cleanroom Products*.

CLEANING THE HORIZONTAL LAMINAR AIRFLOW HOOD

Laminar airflow hoods, also called laminar airflow workbenches (LAFW) are designed to reduce the risk of airborne contamination during the compounding of pharmacological preparations. To ensure proper functioning, the HEPA filter should be inspected and certified every 6 months. Prefilters are changed monthly.

Disinfecting or cleaning the laminar airflow hood is a thorough process that should be completed at the beginning and at the end of your shift. Additional cleaning during your shift may be required after changing from compounding one class of medication to another (ophthalmic solutions to preparation of intravenous admixtures, for example). Also, additional cleaning is required during compounding if there are any spills.

Materials needed are gauze pads or low particle count paper towels, appropriate cleaner approved by infection control at your work site, ETOH (ethyl alcohol) solution, soapy water.

Carefully read through the following steps before performing the task:

- [ ] Turn the laminar flow hood on. The blower should run for 15 to 30 minutes before cleaning/use.
- [ ] First, clean hood by using low-residue cleaner on walls and horizontal surface of hood.
- [ ] Then, squeeze ETOH solution or other appropriate water-based, low-residue cleaner onto walls and horizontal surface of hood.
- [ ] The use of cleaning solutions in the form of a spray is discouraged because the spray may penetrate into the HEPA filters.
- [ ] Use a gauze pad to wipe down the hood. Gauze is preferred over paper towels because gauze has a lower particle count.
- [ ] First, wipe the top of the hood.
- [ ] Next, wipe the rod or pole in the hood.
- [ ] Then, wipe the sides of the hood using an up-and-down motion.
- [ ] Next, wipe the base of the hood.
- [ ] It is important to wipe in a parallel, not circular, motion, working your way from the back of the hood to the front of the hood. Also, work your way from the top of the hood to the bottom.
- [ ] Plexiglas sides should be cleaned with warm, soapy water rather than alcohol.
- [ ] Important to note, never clean or wipe down the HEPA filter grill, which is located on the back panel of the horizontal flow hood.
- [ ] Dispose of soiled gauze pads.

ACTIVITY

Student Directions

1. Review the procedure for cleaning the horizontal laminar airflow hood.
2. Practice the cleaning procedures with your lab partner.
3. Perform the horizontal laminar flow hood cleaning technique for your instructor.

Horizontal Laminar Airflow Hood Cleaning Technique

	YES	NO
Turned on hood and allowed it to run 15-30 minutes		
Properly washed hands		
Properly don an appropriate gown		
Moistened a 4 × 4-inch gauze or other disposable cloth with 70% isopropyl alcohol and wetted down the insides of the hood, including sides and tabletop		
Started from the top right-hand side of the hood, wiped down, across the surface, and up to the top of the left-hand side of the hood		
Moved forward a few inches and repeated the motion in the opposite direction		
Maintained a side-to-side, back-to-front motion		
Previously cleaned surfaces were not contaminated		
Did not clean or spray the HEPA filter or grill		
Did not allow head to enter the hood		
Understood that hood certification is required every six months		
Understood that prefilters must be changed every month		

Student Name _____ Date _____

Lab Partner _____

Grade/Comments _____

_____

Student Comments _____

_____

Horizontal Laminar Airflow Hood

OBJECTIVES

- Gain an awareness of aseptic technique while working with the horizontal laminar airflow hood.

- Evaluate the student's comprehension of aseptic technique in the horizontal laminar airflow hood.

Pre-Lab Information

Shadowing: placement of supplies within the hood that hinders a direct, open path between the filtered airflow and the supply

Critical area: space within the laminar airflow workbench between the HEPA filter and the sterile object

COMPOUNDING: HORIZONTAL LAMINAR AIRFLOW HOOD

The horizontal laminar airflow hood helps reduce the risk of airborne contamination during preparation of sterile products. A constant flow of air moves horizontally across the surface of the work area. The air is filtered with a HEPA (high-efficiency particulate air) filter that removes potentially harmful particles and microorganisms.

The horizontal laminar airflow hood is suitable for nonhazardous drug compounding such as total parenteral nutrition (TPN) solutions.

Pharmacy technician aseptic technique is a critical factor in prevention of contamination during sterile compounding. Review the following workflow steps for sterile compounding technique with a horizontal laminar airflow hood:

☐ Don personal garb.
☐ Use proper hand-washing techniques.
☐ Disinfect laminar flow hood according to procedure listed in Lab 20.
☐ Assemble supplies that will be used in the hood.
☐ Before placing supplies in the hood/workbench, check expiration dating and for indications of defects.
☐ Before placing supplies in the workbench, wipe down the surface of vials and ampules with appropriate disinfectant solution.
☐ When placing supplies in the workbench, be sure to place a distance between each item to eliminate shadowing.
☐ Supplies and objects should be placed at least 6 inches from the sides and front edge of the workbench.
☐ Keep nonessential items out of the hood.
☐ When working in the horizontal laminar airflow hood, hand placement should not obstruct the airflow that moves across the hood, from the back of the workbench to the front of the workbench.

Work with your lab partner in reviewing the aseptic technique for horizontal laminar airflow hood/workbench.

Student Name _____ Date _____

Lab Partner _____

Grade/Comments _____

_____

Student Comments _____

_____

Cleaning the Vertical Airflow Hood

OBJECTIVE

- Demonstrate skills in cleaning the vertical airflow hood/biological safety cabinet.

Pre-Lab Experience

To gain a deeper understanding of pharmaceutical compounding practices, summarize an article on cleanrooms and controlled environments. Select your article from *Controlled Environments Magazine* at www.cemag.us.

Choose from the *Top Stories* on the left side of the home page to search for articles of interest.

CLEANING VERTICAL AIRFLOW HOOD

The vertical airflow hood also may be referred to as a biological safety cabinet (BSC). Air flows in a downward pattern onto the surface of the work area. Most of the air is vented to the outside of the facility, whereas a small amount of the air is recirculated through the filter. The vertical airflow hood is safer to use than a horizontal airflow hood because the air is not blowing directly at the pharmacy technician.

Vertical airflow hoods are grouped into classes depending on the biosafety level of operation of the hood/cabinet. Most vertical airflow hoods are appropriate to use for compounding hazardous agents.

Review the steps for cleaning the vertical laminar airflow hood. Depending on the class of vertical laminar airflow hood/BSC, there may be additional steps in cleaning procedures. Cleaning the BSC differs from cleaning the horizontal laminar airflow hood in that there are additional steps and safety precautions because of the material content of the drug residue.

Vertical Laminar Airflow Hood Cleaning Technique

	YES	NO
Turned on hood and allowed it to run 15-30 minutes		
Properly washed hands		
Properly don an appropriate gown		
Moistened a 4 × 4-inch gauze or other disposable cloth with 70% isopropyl alcohol and wetted down the insides of the hood, including sides and tabletop		
Started from the top right-hand side of the hood, wiped down, across the surface, and up to the top of the left-hand side of the hood		
Moved forward a few inches and repeated the motion in the opposite direction		
Maintained a side-to-side, back-to-front motion		
Previously cleaned surfaces were not contaminated		
Did not clean or spray the HEPA filter or grill		
Understood that hood certification is required every six months		
Understood that prefilters must be changed every month		

Student Name _____ Date _____

Lab Partner _____

Grade/Comments _____

_____

Student Comments _____

_____

Withdrawing Medication from a Vial

OBJECTIVES

- Demonstrate proper technique for withdrawing medication from a vial.

- Label the parts of a syringe and a needle.

Pre-Lab Experience

1. Review the diagram of the parts of the syringe and the needle. After reviewing the diagrams with your lab partner, use a needle and syringe from the classroom lab to demonstrate your understanding of the key components to your instructor.

2. Visit the Becton/Dickinson website to learn more about safety products such as needle shielding systems: *www.bd.com/safety/products/*.

Choose *Pharmaceutical Systems* or *Injection Therapy* from the Products list.

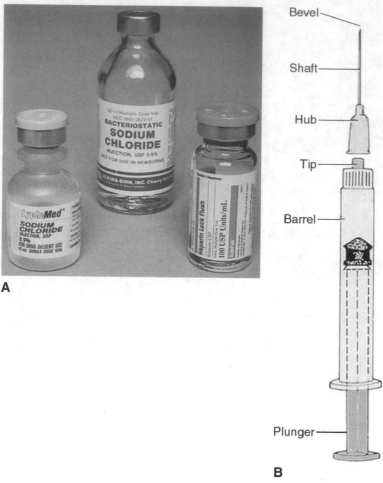

A, Medication in vials. **B,** Parts of a syringe.

WITHDRAWING MEDICATION FROM A VIAL

Injectable medications used for compounding commonly are supplied in a vial. A vial is a plastic or glass container with a rubber closure secured to its top by a metal ring and a metal cover. Follow the steps to review the technique involved for withdrawal of medication from a vial:

☐ Remove cover of vial.
☐ Wipe the rubber surface of the vial with an alcohol swab. Wipe or swab the surface in the same direction with a clean, unused portion of the swab at each wiping motion. Allow the alcohol to dry.
☐ Perform an additional check at this point by comparing the vial to the medication order to ensure that the correct medication is being prepared.
☐ Using your syringe, draw the same volume of air (a few milliliters less) into the syringe as the volume of the drug intended to be drawn from the vial.
☐ Remove the needle from the packaging. Unwrap the paper-covered needles by peeling apart the sides of the package just enough to expose

the needle hub. (Note: Never swab the shaft of the needle because it is coated with silicone.)

- ☐ Attach the needle to the syringe.
- ☐ Uncap the needle.
- ☐ Pierce the rubber closure of the vial with the bevel tip of the needle, bevel side up at a 45-degree angle.
- ☐ Once the rubber surface of the vial has been penetrated, straighten the needle and syringe from 45 degrees to 90 degrees while continuing to insert.
- ☐ Inject the air from the syringe into the vial by putting gentle pressure on the plunger with your thumb.
- ☐ Keeping the needle in the vial, invert the vial and hold it with one hand to control the syringe. Be certain that hand placement does not interrupt clean airflow from the HEPA filter to the needle and vial.
- ☐ Pull back on the plunger of the syringe to draw medication.
- ☐ Draw up the appropriate amount of medication.
- ☐ Read the volume of medication by aligning the outer edge of the plunger with the graduated markings on the syringe.
- ☐ To remove bubbles from the syringe:
  - ☐ Tap the syringe to make the bubbles go to the top of the syringe (toward the needle).
  - ☐ Pull down on the plunger to remove the bubbles, and then push the plunger back to the desired volume.
  - ☐ If air bubbles cannot be tapped free, draw a large air bubble into the syringe and then hold the syringe in a horizontal position and rotate the syringe using the large air bubble to collect smaller ones. Return the syringe to the upright position, and tap the barrel until all air bubbles float to the top.
    Note: Leave the needle in the vial when removing air bubbles.
- ☐ Carefully recap the syringe.

Notify your instructor when you are ready for assessment.

Withdrawing Medication from a Vial

	YES	NO
Turned on the hood and allowed it to run at least 30 minutes before using		
Properly washed hands		
Properly don an appropriate gown		
Applied the appropriate amount of the proper disinfectant/cleanser		
Correctly completed all required calculations before preparing the drug		
Brought all necessary drugs and supplies into the hood prior to preparation, including the medication order, alcohol wipe, vial, needle, and syringe		
Place items in the hood using aseptic technique		
Disinfected gloves		
Compared vial to medication order		
Properly prepared syringe		
Correctly drew medication into syringe		
Accurately read syringe calibrations		
Properly removed bubbles from syringe and recapped it		
Did not contaminate the hood, needle, or syringe during medication preparation		
Ensured that the airflow from the HEPA filter and the air intake grills was not blocked at any time		
Ensured that the outer 6 inches of the hood opening was not used		
Ensured that if hands were withdrawn from the hood, gloves were recleansed before reentering		
Discarded sharps and all other waste properly		

Student Name _____ Date _____

Lab Partner _____

Grade/Comments _____

_____

Student Comments _____

_____

Withdrawing Medication from an Ampule

OBJECTIVES

- Become familiar with the workflow pattern in preparing intravenous products.

- Demonstrate proper technique for withdrawing liquid from an ampule.

Pre-Lab Information

Workflow of Institutional IV Preparation

Workflow varies based on the product being made. Follow these general guidelines:

- Before beginning the act of compounding, review with your pharmacist what amount of antibiotic or other medication will be administered into each intravenous bag.
- After drawing needed medication into the syringe, arrange syringes in the hood.
- Notify your pharmacist that the doses are ready to be checked.
- Only after the pharmacist has checked the syringes should you proceed to combine the medications in the compound.
- The pharmacist will check the final product again before releasing the compounded IV from the pharmacy.

Keep these steps in mind:

- Routine intravenous medications such as antibiotics can be prepared in an assembly-line manner.
- The medication contained in one vial of antibiotic may be used to compound a group of intravenous products. The vial is referred to as a multidose vial.

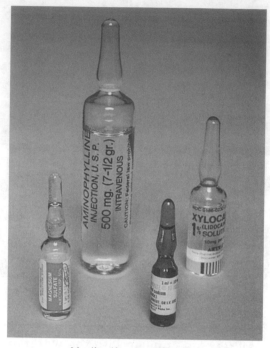

Medication in ampules.

WITHDRAWING MEDICATION FROM AN AMPULE

☐ Perform a check to ensure that the ampule of selected medication matches the medication order.

☐ Before opening the ampule, direct any fluid in the top portion of the ampule to the bottom portion. This may be accomplished by gently tapping the top of the ampule with your finger or by swirling the ampule or by turning the ampule upside down and then quickly flipping the ampule upright.

☐ Use a square of gauze that has been treated with alcohol. Swab the neck of the ampule.

☐ Grasp the top of the glass ampule by wrapping the square of gauze around the neck of the ampule.

☐ Grasp the base of the ampule with your other hand.

☐ Using two hands, snap the ampule top off *away* from you. Make note to open the ampule away from the HEPA filter also (open ampule toward the side of the flow hood).

☐ Assemble the needle and syringe.

☐ Use a filter needle and syringe to draw up the desired amount of liquid from the ampule. Do this by tilting the ampule downward and placing the bevel of the needle inside the bottom corner of the ampule. (A filtered needle is used to prevent small pieces of ampule glass from entering the solution.) Pull all medication out in one draw.

☐ Recap the needle after drawing up the desired amount of fluid and discard the filter needle in a sharps container.

☐ Attach a new capped needle to the syringe and remove air bubbles from syringe.

☐ Use a new needle to inject fluid into medium such as intravenous piggyback.

ACTIVITY

Student Directions

1. With your lab partner, practice opening an ampule.
2. With your lab partner, practice withdrawing fluids from an ampule.
3. Notify your instructor when you are ready for assessment.

Withdrawing Liquid from an Ampule		
	YES	**NO**
Turned on the hood and allowed it to run at least 30 minutes before using		
Properly washed hands		
Properly don an appropriate gown		
Applied the appropriate amount of the proper disinfectant/cleanser		
Correctly completed all required calculations before preparing the drug		
Brought all necessary drugs and supplies into the hood prior to preparation		
Verified that all products are free from contamination or foreign matter		
Removed liquid from ampule tip before opening		
Wiped the neck of the ampule with an alcohol swab before opening		
Used an ampule breaker or wrapped an alcohol pad around ampule neck before opening		
Snapped open the ampule aimed away from you and away from HEPA filters		
Correctly used a filter needle		
Tilted the ampule at an angle to withdraw the appropriate amount of drug, being sure not to fill the syringe to maximum		
Replaced the filter needle with a new needle before transferring the drug to the final container		
The hood, needle, or syringe were not contaminated during medication preparation		
Ensured that the airflow from the HEPA filter and the air intake grills was not blocked at any time		
Ensured that the outer 6 inches of the hood opening was not used		
Ensured that if hands were withdrawn from the hood, gloves were recleansed before reentering		
Discarded sharps and all other waste appropriately		

Student Name _____ Date _____

Lab Partner _____

Grade/Comments _____

_____

Student Comments _____

_____

Reconstituting Dry Powder

OBJECTIVES

- Explain the importance of USP Chapter 797 regulations.

- Successfully demonstrate reconstituting a sterile powder in a vial.

Pre-Lab Experience

USP Chapter 797 applies to health care personnel in all health care facilities where sterile preparations are compounded, stored, and dispensed, including community pharmacies, outsourcing pharmacies, physician practices, infusion clinics, surgical clinics, home care organizations, long-term care facilities, and satellite pharmacies.

Although the addition of USP Chapter 797 is relatively new, the chapter currently is undergoing proposed revisions regarding practice and quality standards.

1. Review USP Chapter 797 regulations at *www.lascoservices.com*.

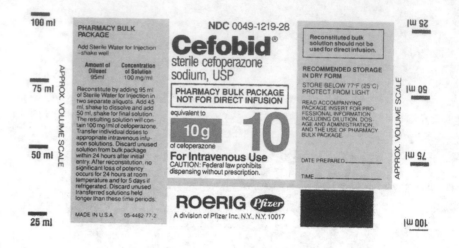

RECONSTITUTING A STERILE POWDER IN A VIAL

Medication may be in a powdered form within a vial. This powdered medication must be reconstituted or made into liquid form before drawing up the medication for compounding sterile preparations.

1. Review the following steps with your lab partner.
2. Notify your instructor when you are ready for assessment.

☐ Read the package instructions that come with the medication. The instructions indicate the type of diluent (diluting agent) to use and the amount of diluent. Following the manufacturer's package instructions is important in order to reconstitute the powder with a compatible liquid.

☐ Place the vial with the powder medication in the flow hood.

☐ Place the vial with the diluent in the flow hood.

☐ When placing vials in the flow hood, be sure there is enough work space between vials to allow for proper handling and no shadowing.

☐ Using the correct technique with the syringe, draw the appropriate amount of diluent.

☐ Avoid recapping the needle used to withdraw diluent.

☐ Using proper technique from previous labs, insert the needle into the powdered vial and add the diluent. As the diluent is added, remove an equal volume of air from the vial. Do this by allowing an equal amount of air to flow back into the syringe from the powder vial. Note: Most powder vials have a vacuum that basically draws the diluent into the vial.

☐ Remove the needle from the vial. (*Note: Pull the plunger back slightly before removing the needle out of the vial. This will help prevent spraying.*)

☐ Discard the syringe and needle into a sharps container.

☐ Mix diluent with powder according to package instructions.

☐ Mixing may involve gently shaking the vial. Or mixing may involve gently turning the vial in the palm of your hands. Another form of mixing is to swirl the vial. Swirling is achieved by holding the vial with your fingertips and making circular-type motions. The latter two ways of mixing alleviate foam and/or bubbles in the final product.

☐ Be certain the drug is dissolved completely and that there is no particulate matter in the solution before proceeding to the next compounding step.

Student Name _____ Date _____

Lab Partner _____

Grade/Comments _____

_____

Student Comments _____

_____

Introducing Liquid into an IV Bag

OBJECTIVES

- Prepare labels for sterile products.

- Demonstrate proper technique of introducing liquid into a PVC bag.

Pre-Lab Experience

Before compounding a preparation, the pharmacist compiles a *master worksheet* detailing the formula, components, compounding directions, sample label, and evaluation and testing requirements of the medication to be compounded.

The pharmacy technician then will work off of a *preparation worksheet* that contains the manufacturer name and lot number and expiration date for each compounding component, date of preparation and personnel involved in preparation, storage requirements, and equipment used during aseptic preparation.

Sterile products should be labeled with the following information:

- Patient name and patient identification
- Control or lot number
- All solution and ingredient names, amount, strength, and concentration (when applicable)
- Expiration date and expiration time if applicable
- Prescribed administration schedule
- Auxiliary labels
- Storage requirements
- Identification of responsible pharmacist and technician
- Any additional information required by state-specific law

The label should be affixed to final container.

1. Practice preparing labels for sterile products.

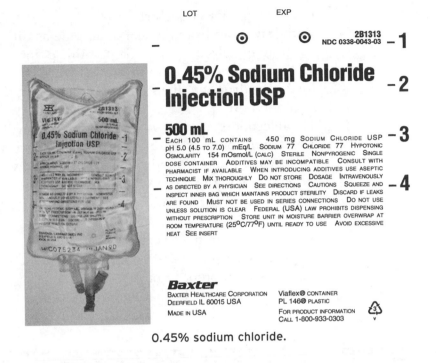

LOT   EXP

2B1313
NDC 0338-0043-03 — **1**

0.45% Sodium Chloride — **2**
Injection USP

500 mL — **3**
Each 100 mL contains 450 mg Sodium Chloride USP
pH 5.0 (4.5 to 7.0) mEq/L Sodium 77 Chloride 77 Hypotonic
Osmolarity 154 mOsmol/L (calc) Sterile Nonpyrogenic Single
dose container Additives may be incompatible Consult with
pharmacist if available When introducing additives use aseptic
technique Mix thoroughly Do not store Dosage Intravenously — **4**
as directed by a physician See directions Cautions Squeeze and
inspect inner bag which maintains product sterility Discard if leaks
are found Must not be used in series connections Do not use
unless solution is clear Federal (USA) law prohibits dispensing
without prescription Store unit in moisture barrier overwrap at
room temperature (25°C/77°F) until ready to use Avoid excessive
heat See insert

Baxter
Baxter Healthcare Corporation   Viaflex® container
Deerfield IL 60015 USA   PL 146® plastic
Made in USA   For product information
                                 Call 1-800-933-0303

0.45% sodium chloride.

INTRODUCING MEDICATION INTO A PLASTIC IV BAG

In previous labs you have practiced the technique of drawing medication from a vial and from an ampule. This lab focuses on the final sterile preparation, which may be compounded in various containers such as plastic bags. Plastic bags are made out of polyvinyl chloride and therefore may be referred to as PVC bags.

Student Directions

1. Review the following compounding steps.
2. Practice the compounding steps with your lab partner.
3. Check off steps when completed.
4. Affix a label to the final product.

☐ Perform aseptic compounding steps as stated in previous labs: proper garb, proper hand washing, laminar flow hood/biological safety cabinet cleaning, gathering of all supplies, and inspection of supplies for expiration dates and any indications of defects. Stop at this point and review aseptic procedures from previous labs.
☐ Perform all calculations before admixture compounding.
☐ Choose the correct IV solution and volume size.
☐ Remove the overwrap from the PVC bag.
☐ Check the PVC bag for leaks by squeezing the bag.
☐ Locate the injection port on the PVC bag. The port is covered by a protective rubber tip.
☐ Position the injection port toward the HEPA filter.

☐ Disinfect the injection port.

☐ Withdraw fluid from the vial or ampule as directed from previous learning in Labs 23 and 24. Stop at this point and review the ampule and vial procedures from previous labs.

☐ Instill the drug into the PVC bag by inserting the needle into the injection port.

☐ The injection port has two diaphragms or partitions that must be pierced: the outer latex tip and an inner plastic partition just inside the port. Avoid puncturing the walls of the bag by entering the port in a straight line with your needle.

☐ Inject the appropriate volume of medication.

☐ Mix the additive well.

☐ Remove air from the PVC bag.

☐ Inspect the final preparation for any particulates.

☐ Label the final preparation.

☐ Notify the pharmacist that the preparation is ready to be checked.

Patient Name	ID #	Room#

☐

Lot #

Solution

Medication Added

Administration Schedule

Expiration Date & Time

Storage Directions   RPh/CPhT

Student Name _____ Date _____

Lab Partner _____

Grade/Comments _____

_____

Student Comments _____

_____

Hazardous Drugs

OBJECTIVES

- Become familiar with guidelines for safe handling of hazardous drugs.

- Become acquainted with nuclear pharmacy.

Pre-Lab Information

MSDS: material safety data sheets; these are details of a hazardous product

Hazardous drug: drug that poses a potential health risk to workers who may be exposed to the drug; drug requires special handling because of the inherent toxicities

Spill kit: readily available kit that contains materials needed to clean up spills of hazardous drugs

PPE: personal protective equipment

Preparation pad: mat or pad placed inside BSC to absorb any leaks or spills

---

HAZARDOUS DRUG SAFETY

Training on site-specific safe handling of hazardous drugs is important because the handling procedures vary according to the hazardous drugs with which you may be working. Regardless of the pharmacy setting in which you are practicing, ask your pharmacy manager for a list of hazardous drugs specific to your site. This lab reviews general guidelines for safe handling of hazardous drugs.

Gloves: Gloves are essential for handling hazardous drugs and must be worn at all times when handling drug vials, performing inventory, and receiving/storing hazardous drugs.

When compounding, double glove and change gloves immediately if they become torn or contaminated.

Receiving: Manufacturers will label totes to indicate the contents of hazardous drugs. Don gloves resistant to hazardous drugs. Be sure to examine the tote and then the drug container for any sign of damage. Do not handle the drugs if there appears to be damage.

Stocking/storage: Hazardous drugs should be separated from other drugs, and the storage shelving of hazardous drugs should be labeled clearly, indicating special handling.

Spill cleanup: Spills occurring in the BSC should be cleaned up immediately. Make use of a spill kit if the volume of the spill exceeds 150 mL or the contents of one drug vial or ampule. Remove broken glass and discard in an appropriate waste container. Thoroughly clean and decontaminate the BSC. Defer use of the BSC if there is spillage onto the HEPA filter. The filter will need to be replaced.

Spills occurring outside of the BSC should be handled by trained personnel only. Each pharmacy site is responsible for policy and procedure on spill cleanup procedures.

Other precautions: When one is transporting hazardous drugs from the pharmacy to the patient care area, the drugs must be packaged in a sealed container. Make note that hazardous drugs should never be sent via pneumatic tubes.

NUCLEAR PHARMACY

The material compounded in nuclear pharmacy has a very short life, or a half-life, of only 6 hours; therefore, nuclear pharmacy sites operate by an on-demand preparation of drugs. Nuclear pharmacy settings practice aseptic technique just as other compounding pharmacy settings. The biggest difference, however, in nuclear pharmacy settings is in time and distance. Time: Pharmacy technicians are trained to work quickly because the less time working with the drug decreases time exposed to the drug. Distance: Tongs are used to handle the syringe, which increases distance between the worker and the drug. Shielding also provides protective distance between the worker and the drug. Syringe shields, for example, are used in the nuclear pharmacy setting.

Nuclear medications may be used for scanning or diagnostic purposes in nuclear medicine clinics.

ACTIVITY

Student Directions

Practice the following steps for hazardous drug vial preparation with your lab partner. Notify your instructor when you are ready for assessment.

Hazardous Drug: Vial Preparation

	YES	NO
Properly washed hands		
Properly don an appropriate gown (chemical gown/double gloves)		
Applied the appropriate amount of the proper disinfectant/cleanser to ensure line clearance		
Was able to locate spill kit		
Was able to locate eye wash station		
Correctly completed all required calculations before preparing the drug		
Properly placed prep mat before preparing drug		
Brought all necessary drugs and supplies into the hood prior to preparation		
Verified that all products are free from contamination or foreign matter		
Properly removed dust covers and cleaned rubber diaphragms		
Accurately inserted needle without coring		
Used proper technique or venting device to prevent drug spraying Did not remove needle from vial until all air bubbles were removed and amount was verified		
Properly removed air bubbles without spilling		
Properly withdrew needle without spilling or aspirating		
Prior to injecting drug, properly cleaned the additive port		
Added drug to final container without coring or puncturing the side of the additive port		
Mixed contents of the container correctly, inspecting for foreign matter		
Always used Luek-Lok syringes and never filled them more than three fourths full		
Before removing the IV container from the hood, properly sealed it in a ziplock bag		
Applied all necessary and appropriate hazardous labels to both product and waste		
Prepared the needle and syringe without contaminating		
Ensured the hood was not contaminated		
Ensured that the airflow from the HEPA filter and the air intake grills was not blocked at any time		
Ensured that the outer 6 inches of the hood opening was not used		
Ensured that if hands were withdrawn from the hood, gloves were recleansed before reentering		
Discarded sharps and all other waste properly		
Removed and discarded gown, gloves, mask, and hair cover appropriately		
Washed hands after removing gloves		

Student Name _____ Date _____

Lab Partner _____

Grade/Comments _____

_____

Student Comments _____

_____

Communication in the Pharmacy

Part I: Nonverbal Communication

OBJECTIVE

- Become conscious of the importance of nonverbal communication.

Pre-Lab Experience

Learn more about listening skills and nonverbal communication skills by greeting a classmate with a handshake. Continue to shake hands for 20-30 seconds. While shaking hands, introduce yourself or tell your classmate a bit about yourself.

Could your classmate repeat the greeting information back to you? What facial expression did each of you have during the greeting?

Describe how the body language and handshake effect the communication exchange.

COMMUNICATION: PART I

Communicating effectively means that you actively listen to what is being said. To understand the meaning of what is being said, the listener must be aware of more than just the spoken word. In the pharmacy setting, when you are talking with a patient or team member, observe body language. Nonverbal communication helps verify that the patient understands directions. As a pharmacy technician, it is important that you display only helpful and concerned nonverbal communications.

1. Test your ability to read nonverbal communications. Log on to *http://nonverbal.ucsc.edu/*.

2. Each title on the website will take you to a different topic on nonverbal communication.
   a. Personal Space
   b. The Human Body
   c. Understanding Cross-Cultural Communication
   d. The Human Face
   e. The Human Voice
3. Answer the questions related to each topic. Return to the main page to access the next topic.

4. List five things you learned about nonverbal communication from other cultures.

Student Name _____ Date _____

Lab Partner _____

Grade/Comments _____

_____

Student Comments _____

_____

Part II: Communication Skills

OBJECTIVES

- Develop on-the-job communication skills.

- Become aware of business telephone etiquette.

Pre-Lab Information

As a pharmacy technician, you will spend much of your day conducting business on the telephone. Every time you make or receive a telephone call at work, you are representing yourself and your pharmacy. The impression you create will be a lasting one. Make sure your voice and mannerism reflect that you are alert and at your best!

1. Answer the phone promptly. Before picking up the receiver, be ready for the call.
2. Identify yourself and your pharmacy name in a clear, friendly voice: "GetWell Pharmacy, this is Susan, how can I help you?"
3. The caller then should identify himself or herself and give a reason for calling. Pronounce the caller's name distinctly and repeat it frequently.
4. Be as helpful as you can. To avoid unnecessary customer delays, handle as much of the call as you can within your scope of practice.
5. If you need to leave the line to obtain information or to refer the call to the pharmacist, it is courteous to give the caller the option of waiting or being called back.

6. Use the hold button when leaving the line so that the caller does not accidentally hear conversations involving protected health information.

Practice telephone etiquette skills with a lab partner.

COMMUNICATION: PART II

Pharmacy technicians communicate every day. Customers that you help depend on your good communication skills in order to have their needs met. Communication involves the ability to express yourself in a way that is clearly understood.

Read the following scenarios and answer the corresponding questions.

Scenario 1

Emma Frances loves to work as a pharmacy technician. She is a favorite among customers for her cheerful attitude and assistance that she offers each one. However, Emma dislikes the inventory/stocking aspects of her job and is often careless about returning stock to the shelf. She returns stock quickly, and other pharmacy personnel find it difficult, if not impossible, to locate stock bottles needed to fill medication orders.

1. What are the potential consequences of Emma's poor quality of work? How would you communicate your concerns to Emma?
   a. For her co-workers?
   b. For her supervising pharmacist?
   c. For her customers?
   d. For her career?

2. How do her actions show a lack of consideration for the pharmacy team as a whole?

Scenario 2

Justin Sweet is a pharmacy technician in the local hospital. Justin likes his schedule, even though often it is hectic, because he is able to take time off work to attend school events for his young daughter. The inpatient pharmacy workload fluctuates depending on patient census. Justin is an educated, certified pharmacy technician. He has an easygoing nature and is well liked by his co-workers. However, at times Justin fails to complete his fill orders for the shift. He is known to leave compounding work in the cleanroom half finished in order to make it to his daughter's game on time.

1. What are the potential consequences of Justin's failure to complete his shift work?
    a. For his co-workers?
    b. For the patients?
    c. For his career?

2. As Justin's co-worker, describe how you would communicate your concerns to him professionally.

Scenario 3

Bernie Hahn is a regular customer at GetWell Pharmacy. She picks up her maintenance medication every month. Usually Bernie is talkative and has a pleasant demeanor. However, when Bernie arrived at the pharmacy this morning, she was short with the cashier and refused counseling on her new heart medication, nifedipine.

1. What are the potential consequences of Bernie's refusal for new drug counseling?

    a. Why might Bernie's mood have been unpleasant when picking up her medication?

    b. As a pharmacy technician, how would you respond to Bernie's mood and her refusal for counseling?

Student Name _____ Date _____

Lab Partner _____

Grade/Comments _____

_____

Student Comments _____

_____

Part III: Communication

OBJECTIVE

Students should realize the following:

- Question assumptions.

- Look beyond the obvious.

- Reject stereotypes.

- Use logic.

- Examine situations from different perspectives.

Pre-Lab Experience

Test your assumptions and prejudices by sharing a photo of a relative or friend with your class. Don't share any other information about your photo.

Find out how accurately your class can guess the following details:

How old is the person?

Does the person have a college degree?

What is the person's occupation?

COMMUNICATION: PART III

Think about a time when your perception was different from someone else's. How do your perceptions influence you while working in the pharmacy?

How do your perceptions influence your life? Can we change the way we perceive things?

View each image. Then write down the first thing you see. After completing the lab, compare your impressions with your lab partner and other classmates.

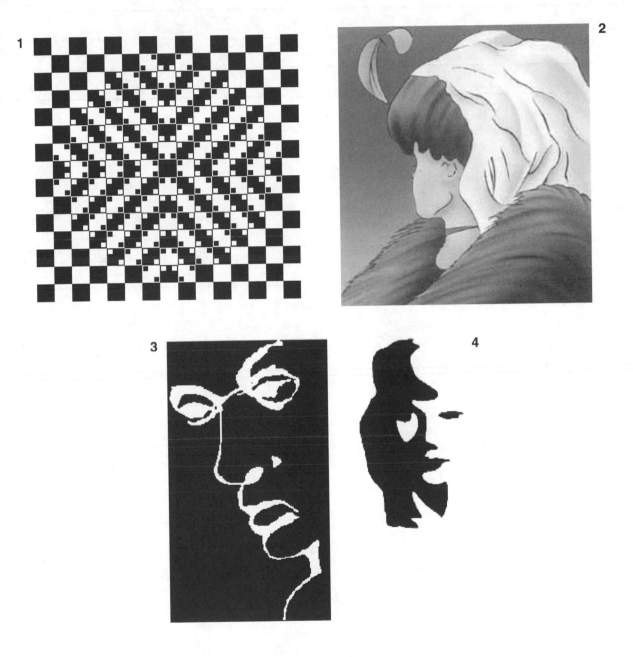

After comparing your images with classmates, you hopefully are able to see two different images within one picture. To be a better communicator, are you able to look beyond your assumptions? Are you able to reject stereotypes that you may have in order to provide better service to your pharmacy customer?

Student Name _____ Date _____

Lab Partner _____

Grade/Comments _____

_____

Student Comments _____

_____

Spanish for the Pharmacy Technician

OBJECTIVES

- Explain pharmacy drive-thru window procedures.

- Communicate pharmacy-specific phrases in Spanish.

Pre-Lab Information

Drive-up Window

The ambulatory pharmacy drive-thru window is used for the convenience of the customer. A customer may choose to use the drive-thru window versus coming into the pharmacy for a variety of reasons. A patient with mobility difficulties may find it convenient to use the drive-thru window, for instance. The difficulty in working with customers at the drive-thru window is that the window is not necessarily a quicker service than coming into the pharmacy store, as viewed by many customers. Insurance claims still need to be processed in the same manner, and filling processes take the same amount of time as if the customer were in the store.

It then becomes the pharmacy technician's responsibility to remind the drive-thru customer pleasantly of the length of wait for prescription processing. Rather than having a customer tie up the window, suggest that the customer return to the drive-thru window in 15 minutes, for instance.

Pharmacy settings sensitive to HIPAA issues are equipped with telephone receivers at the drive-thru window area. By using the telephone receiver located inside the pharmacy, the pharmacy technician can communicate freely with the customer without jeopardizing protected health information. The pharmacy technician is responsible for gathering all pertinent information from the customer as prescriptions are dropped off. As prescriptions are picked up at the window, it is the pharmacy technician's responsibility to offer patient counseling from the pharmacist in charge.

SPANISH FOR THE PHARMACY TECHNICIAN

Twenty-eight million persons in the United States speak Spanish. Spanish is the second most spoken language in the United States. Therefore, it is necessary to become familiar with common Spanish sigs and phrases that are used in the pharmacy.

Also important is the realization of cultural differences. The quality of the patient-pharmacy interaction has an impact on the ability of patients to communicate to their pharmacy and to adhere to treatment. The interaction also has an impact on the patient's feelings about being respected (or disrespected) as an individual, a member of a family, and a member of a cultural group. Your pharmacy employer, co-workers, and patients will appreciate your knowledge of the Spanish culture and language.

Common Spanish Sigs

Take one tablet by mouth every day	TOME 1 TABLETA DIARIA
Take one tablet by mouth every morning	TOME 1 TABLETA DIARIA EN LA MANANA
Take one tablet by mouth every evening	TOME 1 TABLETA DIARIA EN LA NOCHE
Take one capsule by mouth every day	TOME 1 CAPSULA DIARIA
Take one capsule by mouth 2 times a day	TOME 1 CAPSULA DOS VECES AL DIA
Take 1 teaspoonful by mouth every day	TOME 1 CUCHARIADITA (5 mL) DIARIA
Take 1 tablespoonful by mouth every day	TOME 1 CUCHARADA (15 mL) DIARIA

Student Directions

Practice these common pharmacy-specific phrases with a lab partner.

1. What is your name?
   ¿Cuál es su nombre?
   (kwahl ehs soo *nohm*-breh)
2. What is your date of birth?
   ¿Cuál es su fecha de nacimiento?
   (kwahl ehs soo *feh*-chah deh nah-see-mee-*ehn*-toh)
3. Are you allergic to any medicine?
   ¿Es usted alérgico a algunas medicinas?
   (ehs oo-*stehd* ah-*lehr*-hee-koh ah ahl-*goon*-ahs meh-dee-*see*-nahs)
4. The prescription is ready.
   La receta está lista.
   (lah reh-*seh*-tah ehs-*tah lee*-stah)
5. I do not understand.
   Yo no comprendo.
   (yoh noh kohm-*prehn*-doh)

6. Do you have any questions?
   ¿Tiene usted algunas preguntas?
   (tee-*eh*-neh oo-*stehd* ahl-*goo*-nahs preh-*goon*-tahs)
7. Do you need counseling on your medicine?
   ¿Necesita usted aconsejando en su medicina?
   (neh-seh-*see*-tah oo-*stehd* ah-kohn-seh-*hahn*-doh ehn soo
   meh-dee-*see*-nah)

Students Directions

Examine your cultural competence by taking the Culture Quiz. The purpose of this quiz is to stimulate your thinking about cultural differences. Reflect on the quiz questions and answers after completion.

CULTURE QUIZ

1. Cross-cultural misunderstandings between providers and patients can lead to mistrust and frustration but are unlikely to have an impact on objectively measured clinical outcomes.
   a. True
   b. False
2. When the patient and provider come from different cultural backgrounds, the medical history obtained may not be accurate.
   a. True
   b. False
3. When a provider expects that a patient will understand a condition and follow a regimen, the patient is more likely to do so than if the provider has doubts about the patient.
   a. True
   b. False
4. A really conscientious health provider can eliminate his or her own prejudices or negative assumptions about certain types of patients.
   a. True
   b. False
5. When taking a medical history from a patient with a limited ability to speak English, which of the following is LEAST useful?
   a. Asking questions that require the patient to give a simple "yes" or "no" answer, such as "Do you have trouble breathing?" or "Does your knee hurt?"
   b. Encouraging the patient to give a description of his or her medical situation and beliefs about health and illness.
   c. Asking the patient whether he or she would like to have a qualified interpreter for the medical visit.
   d. Asking the patient questions such as, "How has your condition changed over the past two days?" or "What makes your condition get better or worse?"

6. During a medical interview with a patient from a different cultural background, which is the LEAST useful technique?
   a. Asking questions about what the patient believes about her or his illness: what caused the illness, how severe it is, and what type of treatment is needed.
   b. Gently explaining which beliefs about the illness are not correct.
   c. Explaining the "Western" or "American" beliefs about the patient's illness.
   d. Discussing differences in beliefs without being judgmental.

7. When a patient is not adhering to a prescribed treatment after several visits, which of the following approaches is NOT likely to lead to adherence?
   a. Involving family members.
   b. Repeating the instructions very loudly and several times to emphasize the importance of the treatment.
   c. Agreeing to a compromise in the timing or amount of treatment.
   d. Spending time listening to discussions of folk or alternative remedies.

8. When a patient who has not adhered to a treatment regimen states that he or she cannot afford the medications prescribed, it is appropriate to assume that financial factors are indeed the real reasons and not to explore the situation further.
   a. True
   b. False

9. Which of the following are the correct ways to communicate with a patient through an interpreter?
   a. Making eye contact with the interpreter when you are speaking, then looking at the patient while the interpreter is telling the patient what you said.
   b. Speaking slowly, pausing between words.
   c. Asking the interpreter to explain further the patient's statement in order to get a more complete picture of the patient's condition.
   d. None of the above.

10. If a family member speaks English as well as the patient's native language and is willing to act as interpreter, this is the best possible solution to the problem of interpreting.
    a. True
    b. False

11. Which of the following statements is TRUE?
    a. Persons who speak the same language have the same culture.
    b. The people living on the African continent share the main features of African culture.
    c. Cultural background, diet, and religious and health practices, as well as language, can differ widely within a given country or part of a country.
    d. An alert provider usually can predict a patient's health behaviors by knowing from what country he or she comes.

12. Which of the following statements is NOT TRUE?
    a. Friendly (nonsexual) physical contact is an important part of communication for many Latin American people.
    b. Many Asian people think it is disrespectful to ask questions of a health provider.
    c. Most African people are Christian or follow a traditional religion.
    d. Eastern Europeans are highly diverse in terms of customs, language, and religion.

13. Which of the following statements is NOT TRUE?
    a. The incidence of complications of diabetes, including lower-limb amputations and end-stage renal disease, among the black population is double that of whites.
    b. Japanese men who migrate to the United States retain their low susceptibility to coronary heart disease.
    c. Hispanic women have a lower incidence of breast cancer than the majority population.
    d. Some Native Americans/American Indians and Pacific Islanders have the highest rate of type 2 diabetes mellitus in the world.

14. Because Hispanics have a lower incidence of certain cancers than the majority of the U.S. population, their mortality rate from these diseases is correspondingly lower.
    a. True
    b. False

15. Minority and immigrant patients in the United States who go to traditional healers and use traditional medicines generally avoid conventional Western treatments.
    a. True
    b. False

16. Providers whose patients are mostly white, U.S.-born, and middle class still need to know about health practices from different world cultures.
    a. True
    b. False

17. Which of the following is good advice for a provider attempting to use and interpret nonverbal communication?
    a. The provider should recognize that a smile may express unhappiness or dissatisfaction in some cultures.
    b. To express sympathy, a health care provider can touch a patient's arm lightly or pat the patient on the back.
    c. If a patient will not make eye contact with a health care provider, it is likely that the patient is hiding the truth.
    d. When there is a language barrier, the provider can use hand gestures to bridge the gap.

18. Some symbols—a positive nod of the head, a pointing finger, a "thumbs-up" sign—are universal and can help bridge the language gap.
    a. True
    b. False

19. Out of respect for a patient's privacy, the provider should always begin a relationship by seeing an adult patient alone and drawing the family in as needed.
   a. True
   b. False

20. In some cultures, it may be appropriate for female relatives to ask the husband of a pregnant woman to sign consent forms or to explain to him the suggested treatment options if the patient agrees and this is legally permissible.
   a. True
   b. False

21. Which of the following is NOT TRUE of an organization that values cultural competence?
   a. The organization employs or has access to professional interpreters that speak all or at least most of the languages of its clients.
   b. The organization posts signs in different languages and has patient education materials in different languages.
   c. The organization tries to hire staff that mirror the ethnic and cultural mix of its clients.
   d. The organization assumes that professional medical staff do not need to be reminded to treat all patients with respect.

22. A female Muslim patient may avoid eye contact and/or physical contact because _____.
   a. She does not want to spread germs.
   b. Muslim women are taught to be submissive.
   c. Modesty is important in Islamic tradition.
   d. She does not like the provider.

23. Which of the following statements is NOT TRUE?
   a. Diet is an important part of Islam and Hinduism.
   b. North African countries have health care systems that suffer because of political problems.
   c. Arab people historically have not had an impact on the medical field.

Student Name _____ Date _____

Lab Partner _____

Grade/Comments _____

_____

Student Comments _____

_____

Ethics and Law

Ethics

OBJECTIVE

- List principles of the Code of Ethics for Pharmacy Technicians.

Pre-Lab Information

Code of Ethics for Pharmacy Technicians

Preamble
Pharmacy technicians are health care professionals who assist pharmacists in providing the best possible care for patients. The principles of this code, which apply to pharmacy technicians working in all settings, are based on the application and support of the moral obligations that guide all in the pharmacy profession in relationships with patients, health care professional, and society.

Principles

1. A pharmacy technician's first consideration is to ensure the health and safety of the patient and to use knowledge and skills most capably in serving others.
2. A pharmacy technician supports and promotes honesty and integrity in the profession, which includes a duty to observe the law, maintain the highest moral and ethical conduct at all times, and uphold the ethical principles of the profession.
3. A pharmacy technician assists and supports the pharmacist in the safe, efficacious, and cost-effective distribution of health services and health care resources.

Pre-Lab Experience—cont'd

4. A pharmacy technician respects and values the abilities of pharmacist, colleagues, and other health care professionals.
5. A pharmacy technician maintains competency in practice and continually enhances professional knowledge and expertise.
6. A pharmacy technician respects and supports the patient's individuality, dignity, and confidentiality.
7. A pharmacy technician respects the confidentiality of a patient's records and discloses pertinent information only with proper authorization.
8. A pharmacy technician never assists in the dispensing, promoting, or distribution of medications or medical devices that are not of good quality or do not meet the standards required by law.
9. A pharmacy technician does not engage in any activity that will discredit the profession, and will expose, without fear or favor, illegal or unethical conduct in the profession.
10. A pharmacy technician associates and engages in the support of organizations that promote the profession of pharmacy through the use and enhancement of pharmacy technicians.

ETHICS

Ethics are concerned with standards of behavior and the concept of right and wrong, over and above the legal restrictions. A code of ethics governs behavior and increases the level of competence and standard of care within a group. The pharmacy profession has a code of ethics. An illegal act by a pharmacy technician is always unethical, but an unethical act is not necessarily illegal.

Read the following case studies and answer the corresponding questions.

Case 1

J. B., Individually and as Special
Administratrix of the Estate of C. H. B., Deceased
Plaintiff,
vs
Dr. David McNeil, Dr. Darryl L. Pure, Ph.D.,
and Eli Lilly and Company,
Defendants.

In her 10-year-old malpractice and Prozac liability lawsuit refiled on January 27, 1999, Mrs. B. claimed, among many other things, that at various times during 1991, psychiatrist McNeil negligently prescribed Prozac and various other medications without properly monitoring her bipolar husband who had previously attempted suicide and that psychologist Pure also failed to diagnose him correctly and also directed his psychotherapy toward the treatment of dysthymia instead of bipolar disorder.

Against Eli Lilly she claimed, among many other things, that Eli Lilly misled the Food and Drug Administration to obtain approval for Prozac, failed to disclose full results of research and testing related to it, failed to warn or adequately warn about the extent of risks to certain persons to whom Prozac was prescribed, failed to inform the FDA and doctors who would prescribe it, that before 1991, the German government required a warning with the prescribing information for Prozac that it should be used with particular caution in persons who are suicidal or agitated and that a concomitant sedative be used to counteract the stimulating effects of Prozac.

1. If the patient, Mr. B., is injured through no fault of yours, could you still be ethically responsible?

2. Do you feel the manufacturer, Eli Lilly, is liable? Is the psychiatrist McNeil negligent?

Case 2

Class Action Pharmacy Lawsuit Case

Urgent Care Pharmacy located in Spartanburg, South Carolina, is suspected of producing a contaminated steroid pain injection that so far has caused three persons to contract fungal meningitis, one of whom has died.

State and federal health authorities believe the injections may have been contaminated with the fungus *Wangiella dermatitidis* during their production. The tainted drugs then were shipped to pain clinics in five states, including North Carolina. The North Carolina clinics were located in Jacksonville, Pinehurst, and Goldsboro.

Please note: Complaints about pharmacists, pharmacies, and other entities registered by the State Board of Pharmacy are handled through administrative proceedings required by law. These proceedings are not equivalent to a trial in court. The Board of Pharmacy takes action based upon the files and records brought before it. Court review of its decisions may occur at a later time.

1. Do you consider there to be any moral obligations for the pharmacy technician according to the principles listed in the current code of ethics?

Case 3

Internet pharmacy practice has exploded within the past few years. Patients look to the World Wide Web to shop for hassle-free, convenient prescriptions.

Online consultations often involve the patient completing an online question-naire, rather than receiving a traditional physical exam by a physician. Although online consultations cannot take the place of a traditional exam, they do enable patients to receive medication for conditions that, in many circumstances, do not actually require a physical exam.

Highly trained and qualified pharmacists provide you with the high standards of pharmaceutical care. All medicines provided are obtained from legitimate pharmaceutical wholesalers or in some cases directly from the manufacturer. In this way you can be sure that you receive at all times the same quality medication that you would receive from your neighborhood drugstore.

1. In general, are Internet pharmacies able to enforce standards of protection for patients?

2. Do you feel the patient's privacy rights are in jeopardy when transferring prescription information over the Internet?

Case 4

Overworked and Error-Prone Pharmacist Misfills Prescription: Confidential Settlement

The plaintiff began to experience high blood pressure, weight loss, extreme headaches, uncontrollable diarrhea, blurred vision, and changes in her mental state in April 1999. Her treating physician was unable to diagnose the cause of her illness—and in particular could not understand why the patient's blood pressure medication that he had prescribed, Avapro, was no longer working.

One month later, the plaintiff noticed that the contents of her medication bottle were listed as Avara, a rheumatoid arthritis drug. She telephoned the national pharmacy chain where she had picked up her prescription, but she was not able to speak to the pharmacist who filled the order. The plaintiff discovered that the night pharmacist who had filled the plaintiff's medication had misfilled 45 prescriptions between June 1997 and November 2000 at that pharmacy. Other pharmacists at this same store averaged one error per year. The plaintiff also discovered that the defendant pharmacist frequently worked 10-hour shifts 7 nights in a row.

After the error in this case became known to his supervisor, the pharmacist was transferred to a different pharmacy in another town. But the regional supervisor did not tell his new on-site supervisor about his pattern of errors. The district supervisor also disclosed during discovery that she had never fired a pharmacist for incompetence, and she has been with the company since 1994. The plaintiff also discovered that the pharmacy does not have a nationwide written policy requiring prescription misfills to be tracked.

According to a published account, after the plaintiff filed a negligence case in district court, a confidential settlement was reached shortly before trial.

1. Was it appropriate to transfer the pharmacy supervisor to a different pharmacy location?

2. Is there a violation of the Code of Ethics for Pharmacy Technicians?

3. Read about professional liability insurance programs for pharmacy technicians and other health care providers by visiting Healthcare Providers Service Organization at *www.hpso.com*.

Student Name _____ Date _____

Lab Partner _____

Grade/Comments _____

_____

Student Comments _____

_____

Law

OBJECTIVE

- List the responsibilities of pharmacy technicians as they apply to state-specific regulations.

Pre-Lab Experience

Review your state-specific pharmacy technician restrictions, guidelines, powers, and duties. Commit these pharmacy technician state regulations to memory. Your instructor will provide you with a copy of current regulations. You also may view state pharmacy law by logging onto *www.ptcb.org*. You also may view state pharmacy law by logging onto your State Board of Pharmacy website.

PHARMACY LAW

In each state, the state board of pharmacy administers state regulations for the practice of pharmacy. Following state-specific regulations is mandatory. You also must know the regulations of your own state, because each state differs on aspects of pharmacy practice.

State Regulations

1. Log onto the National Association of Boards of Pharmacy website at *www.nabp.net*.

2. Click on the *Boards of Pharmacy* tab to access your State Board of Pharmacy website.
3. Access pharmacy technician regulations in your state.
4. Answer the following questions regarding your state pharmacy law.

QUESTIONS FOR REVIEW

1. May a pharmacy technician in the hospital/institutional setting accept called-in prescriptions from a physician's office? In the community setting?

2. May a pharmacy technician in the hospital/institutional setting enter a prescription into the pharmacy computer? In the community setting?

3. May a pharmacy technician in the hospital/institutional setting check another pharmacy technician's work? In the community setting?

4. May a pharmacy technician in the hospital/institutional setting call a physician for refill authorization? In the community setting?

5. May a pharmacy technician in the hospital/institutional setting compound medications for dispensing? In the community setting?

6. May a pharmacy technician in the hospital/institutional setting transfer prescriptions via the telephone? In the community setting?

7. Is the pharmacy technician required to be licensed in your state? Certified? Registered?

8. What is the ratio of pharmacy technicians to pharmacists in your state?

9. List three functions a pharmacy technician may *not* perform in your state.
   a.
   b.
   c.

Student Name _____ Date _____

Lab Partner _____

Grade/Comments _____

_____

Student Comments _____

_____

Essential Technician Skills and Drug Product Knowledge

Over-the-Counter Labels

OBJECTIVE

- List the information that must appear on an over-the-counter medication label.

Pre-Lab Experience

Medication labeling is an important aspect in patient compliance. Ideally, patients who are using an OTC product should understand dosing directions for that product by information provided on the product label.

Medication labeling is also an important aspect of safety standards. What changes would you make to the manufacturer's labeling to promote safe medication practices?

Choose two over-the-counter products from your classroom lab. Describe the improvements that you would make to the product labeling and/or packaging.

OVER-THE-COUNTER LABELING

Standardized labeling for OTC drug products is intended to make it easier for consumers to read and understand OTC drug products. The new *OTC Drug Facts Label* uses simple language and an easy to read format to help individuals compare and select OTC medications.

The following information must appear on the OTC label in this order:

- The active ingredients of the product
  - Including the amount of active ingredient in each dosage
- The purpose of the medication
- The uses or indications for the medication
- Specific warnings
  - Warnings include when the product should not be used
  - Warnings include when to consult a physician or pharmacist
  - Warning section describes side effects that could occur
  - Warning section includes substances or activities to avoid
- Dosage instructions addressing when, how, and how often to take medication
- The inactive ingredients of the product

QUESTIONS FOR REVIEW

Refer to the OTC label on p. 147. Answer the following questions:

1. What is the active ingredient in this medication?

2. *"Ask a doctor before use if you have glaucoma"* is listed under what OTC label category?

3. Regarding the dosage instructions: *When* should the medicine be taken? *How* should the medicine be taken? *How often* should the medicine be taken?

4. Does this OTC label comply with labeling regulations? Explain.

Drug Facts

Active ingredient (in each tablet)   **Purpose**
Chlorpheniramine maleate 2 mg . . . . Antihistamine

Uses temporarily relieves these symptoms due to hay fever or other upper respiratory allergies;
■ sneezing   ■ runny nose   ■ itchy, watery eyes   ■ itchy throat

---

Warnings

Ask a doctor before use if you have
■ glaucoma   ■ a breathing problem such as emphysema or chronic bronchitis
■ trouble urinating due to an enlarged prostate gland

Ask a doctor or pharmacist before use if you are taking tranquilizers or sedatives

---

When using this product
■ you may get drowsy   ■ avoid alcoholic drinks
■ alcohol, sedatives, and tranqulilzers may increase drowsiness
■ be careful when driving a motor vehicle or operating machinery
■ excitability may occur, especially in children

If pregnant or breast-feeding, ask a health professional before use.
Keep out of reach of children. In case of overdose, get medical help or contact a Poison Control Center right away.

Directions

adults and children 12 years and over	take 2 tablets every 4 to 6 hours; not more than 12 tablets in 24 hours
children 6 years to under 12 years	take 1 tablet every 4 to 6 hours; not more than 6 tablets in 24 hours
children under 6 years	ask a doctor

Other information store at 20–25 °C (68–77 °F) ■ protect from excessive moisture

---

Inactive ingredients D&C yellow no. 10, lactose, magnesium stearate, microcrystalline cellulose, pregelatinized starch

---

Weight Conversions

GRAINS	DRAMS	OUNCES	POUNDS	MILLIGRAMS	GRAMS	SCRUPLES	KILOGRAMS
1				65			
20					1.3	1	
60	1					3	
480	8	1			30		
		16	1		454		
			2.2				1

Capacity Conversions

MINIMS	FLUID DRAMS	FLUID OUNCES	PINTS	QUARTS	GALLONS	MILLILITERS
60	1	0.002				0.06
480	8	1				30
		16	1			480
		32	2	1		
			8	4	1	

Household Measure Conversions

TEASPOONFULS	TABLESPOONFULS	DRAMS	FLUID OUNCES	MILLILITERS	DROPS
1		1	0.167	5	80 (approximate)
3	1	4	0.5	15	

Student Name _____ Date _____

Lab Partner _____

Grade/Comments _____

_____

Student Comments _____

_____

Design a Drug

OBJECTIVES

- Indicate consumer information required on over-the-counter medication labels.

- Differentiate safe medication practices in labeling.

Pre-Lab Experience

In the United States, the Food and Drug Administration (FDA) must approve new medications before marketing. The approval process can be lengthy and costly to the manufacturer. The goal of the FDA is to determine whether the proposed medication is safe and effective in its proposed use. Another function of the FDA is to determine whether the proposed labeling of the medication is appropriate. The FDA also investigates whether the manufacturing methods are adequate in preserving the strength, quality, purity, and identity of the medication.

1. Access the Center for Drug Evaluation and Research website at *www.fda.gov/drugs/default.htm*.

2. Read about the FDA drug review process: *From Fish to Pharmacies: The Story of a Drug's Development* at www.fda.gov/drugs/ developmentapprovalprocess/howdrugsaredevelopedandapproved/ default.htm.

3. Review the article attached to this lab, *The FDA's Drug Review Process: Ensuring Drugs Are Safe and Effective,* by Michelle Meadows.

DESIGN-A-DRUG

What would it be like to have an antigravity medication available that enables you to fly? How about a transdermal patch that, when applied, allows you to be transported to any destination you want?

Use your imagination to design a fantasy drug. This new medication can be completely fictional or based on curing a real disease.

1. Design a poster advertising your new medication.
   a. You may use cutouts from old magazines, computer clip art, or your own artwork. Be creative!
2. Include all of the consumer information required on OTC manufacturers' labels.
   a. Refer to Lab 32 to review information needed.

Student Name _____ Date _____

Lab Partner _____

Grade/Comments _____

_____

Student Comments _____

_____

THE FDA'S DRUG REVIEW PROCESS: ENSURING DRUGS ARE SAFE AND EFFECTIVE[1]

Michelle Meadows

The path a drug travels from a lab to your medicine cabinet is usually long, and every drug takes a unique route. Often, a drug is developed to treat a specific disease. An important use of a drug may also be discovered by accident.

For example, Retrovir (zidovudine, also known as AZT) was first studied as an anti-cancer drug in the 1960s with disappointing results. It wasn't until the 1980s that researchers discovered the drug could treat AIDS, and the Food and Drug Administration approved the drug, manufactured by GlaxoSmithKline, for that purpose in 1987.

Most drugs that undergo pre-clinical (animal) testing never even make it to human testing and review by the FDA. The drugs that do must undergo the agency's rigorous evaluation process, which scrutinizes everything about the drug—from the design of clinical trials to the severity of side effects to the conditions under which the drug is manufactured.

Stages of Drug Development and Review

1. INVESTIGATIONAL NEW DRUG APPLICATION (IND)

The FDA first enters the picture when a drug sponsor submits an IND to the agency. Sponsors—companies, research institutions, and other organizations that take responsibility for marketing a drug—must show the FDA results of pre-clinical testing they've done in laboratory animals and what they propose to do for human testing. At this stage, the FDA decides whether it is reasonably safe to move forward with testing the drug on humans.

2. CLINICAL TRIALS

Drug studies in humans can begin only after an IND is reviewed by the FDA and a local institutional review board (IRB). The board is a panel of scientists and non-scientists in hospitals and research institutions that oversees clinical research.

IRBs approve the clinical trial protocols, which describe the type of people who may participate in the clinical trial, the schedule of tests and procedures, the medications and dosages to be studied, the length of the study, the study's objectives, and other details. IRBs make sure the study is acceptable, that participants have given consent and are fully informed of their risks, and that researchers take appropriate steps to protect patients from harm.

Phase 1 studies are usually conducted in healthy volunteers. The goal here is to determine what the drug's most frequent side effects are and, often, how the drug is metabolized and excreted. The number of subjects typically ranges from 20 to 80.

Phase 2 studies begin if Phase 1 studies don't reveal unacceptable toxicity. While the emphasis in Phase 1 is on safety, the emphasis in Phase 2 is on effectiveness. This phase aims to obtain preliminary data on whether the drug works in people who have a certain disease or condition. For controlled trials, patients receiving the drug are compared with similar patients receiving a different treatment—usually a placebo or a different drug. Safety continues to be evaluated, and short-term side effects are studied. Typically, the number of subjects in Phase 2 studies ranges from a few dozen to about 300.

Phase 3 studies begin if evidence of effectiveness is shown in Phase 2. These studies gather more information about safety and effectiveness, studying different populations and different dosages and using the drug in combination with other drugs. The number of subjects usually ranges from several hundred to about 3,000 people.

Phase 4 studies occur after a drug is approved. They may explore such areas as new uses or new populations, long-term effects, and how participants respond to different dosages.

3. NEW DRUG APPLICATION (NDA)

This is the formal step a drug sponsor takes to ask that the FDA consider approving a new drug for marketing in the United States. An NDA includes all animal and human data and analyses of the data, as well as information about how the drug behaves in the body and how it is manufactured.

When an NDA comes in, the FDA has 60 days to decide whether to file it so that it can be reviewed. The FDA can refuse to file an application that is incomplete. For example, some required studies may be missing. In accordance with the Prescription Drug User Fee Act (PDUFA), the FDA's Center for Drug Evaluation and Research (CDER) expects to review and act on at least 90 percent of NDAs for standard drugs no later than 10 months after the applications were received. The review goal is six months for priority drugs. (See "The Role of User Fees.")

The Tufts Center for the Study of Drug Development in Boston estimates that about 1 in 5 drugs that enter clinical testing ultimately are approved by the FDA.

How often the FDA meets with a drug sponsor varies, but the two most common meeting points are at the end of Phase 2 clinical trials and pre-NDA—right before a new drug application is submitted.

At the end of Phase 2, the FDA and sponsors try to come to an agreement on how the large-scale studies in Phase 3 should be done. The pre-NDA meeting is for discussing what the FDA expects to see in the application.

There is also continuous interaction throughout the review process. For example, over roughly six years, the sponsor Merck Research Laboratories of West Point, Pa., and the FDA had a half-dozen face-to-face meetings and about 28 teleconferences regarding the asthma drug Singulair (montelukast sodium).

In 1992, Merck submitted an IND for Singulair so that it could begin conducting studies in humans. After clinical trials were complete, the company submitted a new drug application in February 1997. The FDA approved Singulair in February 1998.

"It's the clinical trials that take so long—usually several years," says Sandra Kweder, M.D., deputy director for the Office of New Drugs in CDER. "The emphasis on speed for FDA mostly relates to review time and timelines of being able to meet with sponsors during a drug's development," she says.

Reviewing Applications

Though FDA reviewers are involved with a drug's development throughout the IND stage, the official review time is the length of time it takes to review a new drug application and issue an action letter, an official statement informing a drug sponsor of the agency's decision.

Once a new drug application is filed, an FDA review team—medical doctors, chemists, statisticians, microbiologists, pharmacologists, and other experts—evaluates whether the studies the sponsor submitted show that the drug is safe and effective for its proposed use. No drug is absolutely safe; all drugs have side effects. "Safe" in this sense means that the benefits of the drug appear to outweigh the risks.

The review team analyzes study results and looks for possible problems with the application, such as weaknesses of the study design or analyses. Reviewers determine whether they agree with the sponsor's results and conclusions, or whether they need any additional information to make a decision.

Each reviewer prepares a written evaluation containing conclusions and recommendations about the application. These evaluations are then considered by team leaders, division directors, and office directors, depending on the type of application.

Steven Hirschfeld, M.D., Ph.D., a medical officer in CDER's Division of Oncology Drug Products, says, "It is impossible to have all the information we wish to have at the time we need it." One factor is the practical size of clinical trials, which typically include several thousand subjects at the most.

"We are using information about past experience from a select group of people—those enrolled in particular clinical trials—and attempting to predict the future experience of the population at large."

For Hirschfeld, recognizing uncertainty and attempting to minimize it is one of the greatest challenges in reviewing information about health products. Recommending designs for clinical trials is one way to ask for more information and resolve unanswered questions, he says. Controlled clinical trials allow the FDA to conclude whether a new drug has shown substantial evidence of safety and effectiveness.

In Hirschfeld's opinion, some aspects of the job are similar to the responsibilities of air traffic controllers in the sense that they also analyze information that's available to them and make recommendations that can be acted on.

"People bringing planes in have to balance weather, other planes in the sky, ground traffic, and arrival and departure schedules, all without placing people at greater risk," he says. They can rearrange flight schedules and use different runways to lower the risk of problems, and the FDA can limit a drug's use or take other steps to lower the risk of problems, he says. "We all have responsibilities to protect or guide those who are vulnerable, and we use the best analytic tools at our disposal."

Reviewers receive training that fosters consistency in drug reviews, and good review practices remain a high priority for the agency. For example, CDER recently held a two-day retreat in which clinical reviewers discussed review priorities, including improved communication between drug review divisions in CDER regarding drugs being reviewed for more than one indication.

Sometimes the FDA calls on advisory committees made up of outside experts who help the agency decide on drug applications. Whether an advisory committee is needed depends on many things.

"Some considerations would be if it's a drug that has significant questions, if it's the first in its class, or the first for a given indication," says Mark Goldberger, M.D., director of CDER's office that evaluates drugs to treat infectious diseases and immunosuppressive agents. "Generally, FDA takes the advice of advisory committees, but not always," he says. "Their role is just that—to advise."

Accelerated Approval

Traditional approval requires that clinical benefit be shown before approval can be granted. Accelerated approval is given to some new drugs for serious and life-threatening illnesses that lack satisfactory treatments. This allows an NDA to be approved before measures of effectiveness that would usually be required for approval are available.

Instead, less traditional measures called "surrogate endpoints" are used to evaluate effectiveness. These are laboratory findings or signs that may not be a direct measurement of how a patient feels, functions, or survives, but are considered likely to predict benefit. For example, a surrogate endpoint could be the lowering of HIV blood levels for short periods of time with anti-retroviral drugs.

Gleevec (imatinib mesylate), an oral treatment for patients with a life-threatening form of cancer called chronic myeloid leukemia (CML), received accelerated approval. The drug was also approved under the FDA's orphan drug program, which gives financial incentives to sponsors for manufacturing drugs that treat rare diseases. Gleevec blocks enzymes that play a role in cancer growth. The approval was based on results of three large Phase 2 studies, which showed the drug could substantially reduce the level of cancerous cells in the bone marrow and blood.

The sponsor, Novartis Pharmaceuticals Corp. of East Hanover, N.J., submitted the IND in April 1998. The FDA received the NDA in February 2001, and the drug was approved two and a half months later in May 2001. Novartis has made commitments to conduct Phase 4 studies that investigate Gleevec's clinical benefit, such as increased progression-free survival in the treatment of CML.

Most drugs to treat HIV have been approved under accelerated approval provisions, with the company required to continue its studies after the drug is on the market to confirm that its effects on virus levels are maintained and that it ultimately benefits the patient. Under accelerated approval rules, if studies don't confirm the initial results, the FDA can withdraw the approval.

Because premarket review can't catch all potential problems with a drug, the FDA continues to track approved drugs for adverse events through a postmarketing surveillance program.

Bumps in the Road

If the FDA decides that the benefits of a drug outweigh the risks, the drug will receive approval and can be marketed in the United States. But if there are problems with an NDA, the FDA may decide that a drug is "approvable" or "not approvable."

A designation of approvable means that the drug can probably be approved, provided that some issues are resolved first. This might involve the sponsor and the FDA coming to a final agreement on what should go on the drug's label, for example. It could also involve more difficult issues, such as the adequacy of information on how people respond to various dosages of the drug.

A designation of "not approvable" describes deficiencies significant enough that it is not clear that approval can be obtained in the future, at least not without substantial additional data.

Common problems include unexpected safety issues that crop up or failure to demonstrate a drug's effectiveness. A sponsor may need to conduct additional studies—perhaps studies of more people, different types of people, or for a longer period of time.

Manufacturing issues are also among the reasons that approval may be delayed or denied. Drugs must be manufactured in accordance with standards called good manufacturing practices, and the FDA inspects manufacturing facilities before a drug can be approved. If a facility isn't ready for inspection, approval can be delayed. Any manufacturing deficiencies found would need to be corrected before approval.

"Sometimes a company may make a certain amount of a drug for clinical trials. Then when they go to scale up, they may lose a supplier or end up with quality control issues that result in a product of different chemistry," says the FDA's Kweder. "Sponsors have to show us that the product that's going to be marketed is the same product that they tested."

John Jenkins, M.D., director of CDER's Office of New Drugs, says, "It's often a combination of problems that prevent approval." Close communication with the FDA early on in a drug's development reduces the chance that an application will have to go through more than one cycle of review, he says. "But it's no guarantee."

The FDA outlines the justification for its decision in an action letter to the drug sponsor. When the action is either approvable or not approvable, CDER gives the sponsor a chance to meet with agency officials to discuss the deficiencies. At that point, the sponsor can choose to ask for a hearing or correct any deficiencies and submit new information.

The Role of User Fees

Since the Prescription Drug User Fee Act (PDUFA) was passed in 1992, more than 700 drugs and biologics have come to the market, including new medicines to treat cancer, AIDS, cardiovascular disease, and life-threatening infections. PDUFA has allowed the Food and Drug Administration to bring access to new drugs as fast or faster than anywhere in the world, all while maintaining the same thorough review process.

Under PDUFA, drug companies agree to pay fees that boost FDA resources, and the FDA agrees to time goals for its review of new drug applications. Along with supporting increased staff, drug user fees help the FDA upgrade resources in information technology. The agency has moved toward an electronic submission and review environment, now accepting more electronic applications and filing review documents electronically.

The goals set by PDUFA apply to the review of original new human drug and biological applications, resubmissions of original applications, and supplements to approved applications. The second phase of PDUFA, known as PDUFA II, was reauthorized in 1997 and extended the user fee program through September 2002. PDUFA III, which extends to 2007, was reauthorized in June 2002.

The FDA continues to meet or exceed PDUFA's review goals, which have become more demanding each year. FDA's Center for Drug Evaluation and Research (CDER) approved 66 new drugs in 2001, 24 of which were new molecular entities (NMEs) with ingredients never marketed before in the United States. Ten were priority products, believed to represent an advance over available therapies. The FDA's Center for Biologics Evaluation and Research (CBER) reviewed 16 complex biological license applications (BLAs) last year. Two of the BLAs reviewed were classified as priority products. Biologics are medical products derived from living sources, such as vaccines and blood products.

In addition to setting time frames for review of applications, PDUFA sets goals to improve communication between the FDA and drug sponsors. PDUFA outlines how fast the FDA must respond to requests from sponsors and how often meetings should occur. Throughout a drug's development, the FDA advises sponsors on how to study certain classes of drugs, how to submit data, what kind of data is needed, and how clinical trials should be designed.

The Quality of Clinical Data

The Food and Drug Administration relies on data that sponsors submit to decide whether a drug should be approved. To protect the rights and welfare of people in clinical trials, and to verify the quality and integrity of data submitted, the FDA's Division of Scientific Investigations (DSI) conducts inspections of clinical investigators' study sites. DSI also reviews the records of institutional review boards to be sure they are fulfilling their role in patient protection.

"FDA investigators compare information that clinical investigators provided to sponsors on case report forms with information in source documents such as medical records and lab results," says Carolyn Hommel, a consumer safety officer in DSI.

DSI seeks to determine such things as whether the study was conducted according to the investigational plan, whether all adverse events were recorded, and whether the subjects met the inclusion/exclusion criteria outlined in the study protocol.

At the conclusion of each inspection, FDA investigators prepare a report summarizing any deficiencies. In cases where they observe numerous or serious deviations, such as falsification of data, DSI classifies the inspection as "official action indicated" and sends a warning letter or Notice of Initiation of Disqualification Proceedings and Opportunity to Explain (NIDPOE) to the clinical investigator, specifying the deviations that were found.

The NIDPOE begins an administrative process to determine whether the clinical investigator should remain eligible to receive investigational products and conduct clinical studies.

CDER conducts about 300 to 400 clinical investigator inspections annually. About 3 percent are classified in this "official action indicated" category.

Drug Review Steps

1. Pre-clinical (animal) testing
2. An investigational new drug application (IND) outlines what the sponsor of a new drug proposes for human testing in clinical trials
3. Phase 1 studies (typically involve 20 to 80 people)
4. Phase 2 studies (typically involve a few dozen to about 300 people)
5. Phase 3 studies (typically involve several hundred to about 3,000 people)
6. The pre-NDA period, just before a new drug application (NDA) is submitted; a common time for the FDA and drug sponsors to meet
7. Submission of a new drug application is the formal step asking the FDA to consider a drug for marketing approval
8. After an NDA is received, the FDA has 60 days to decide whether to file it so it can be reviewed
9. If the FDA files the NDA, an FDA review team is assigned to evaluate the sponsor's research on the drug's safety and effectiveness
10. The FDA reviews information that goes on a drug's professional labeling, guidance on how to use the drug
11. The FDA inspects the facilities where the drug will be manufactured as part of the approval process
12. FDA reviewers will approve the drug or find it either "approvable" or "not approvable"

Controlled Drugs

OBJECTIVES

- Discriminate between scheduled classes of controlled substances.

- Indicate DEA forms used by pharmacy personnel.

Pre-Lab Experience

The Food and Drug Administration (FDA) and the Drug Enforcement Administration (DEA) work together to create and update the list of scheduled drugs.

1. Visit the DEA website at *www.dea.gov*.
2. Click on *Drug Scheduling* on the left side of the DEA home page.
3. List five substances named in schedule I. What are the street names of these substances?

SCHEDULED DRUGS

Scheduled drugs also may be referred to as controlled drugs, narcotics, or narcs. Scheduled drugs are prescription drugs that are placed into a scheduled class because they have a potential for abuse because of their addictive properties.

When filling a prescription for schedule II narcotics, rather than using an electronic scale or counting machine, the medication must always be counted by hand. Medication also should be double-counted by a pharmacy technician co-worker.

1. Schedule I
   a. The drug or other substance has a high potential for abuse.
   b. The drug or other substance currently has no accepted medical use in treatment in the United States.
   c. There is a lack of accepted safety for use of the drug or other substance under medical supervision.
2. Schedule II
   a. The drug or other substance has a high potential for abuse.
   b. The drug or other substance currently has an accepted medical use in treatment in the United States or a currently accepted medical use with severe restrictions.
   c. Abuse of the drug or other substances may lead to severe psychological or physical dependence.

   No controlled substance in schedule II that is a prescription drug as determined under the Federal Food, Drug, and Cosmetic Act may be dispensed without the written prescription of a practitioner, except that in emergency situations, such drug may be dispensed on oral prescription in accordance with written law. No prescription for a controlled substance in schedule II may be refilled.
   d. Warning on label: The label of a drug listed in schedule II, III, or IV shall, when dispensed to or for a patient, contain a clear, concise warning that it is a crime to transfer the drug to any person other than the patient.
   e. Storage/record keeping: Special record keeping is required of schedule II narcotics. Many pharmacies keep a log book of perpetual inventory. Also, some pharmacies may keep the schedule II narcotics in a separate, more isolated area of the pharmacy. Much of the time the narcotics are stored in a locked area.
3. Schedule III
   a. The drug or other substance has a potential for abuse less than the drugs or other substances in schedules I and II.
   b. The drug or other substance currently has an accepted medical use in treatment in the United States.
   c. Abuse of the drug or other substance may lead to moderate or low physical dependence or high psychological dependence.

   No controlled substance in schedule III or IV that is a prescription drug as determined under the Federal Food, Drug, and Cosmetic Act may be dispensed without a written or oral prescription. Such prescriptions may not be filled or refilled more than 6 months after the date thereof or be refilled more than 5 times after the date of the prescription unless renewed by the practitioner.
4. Schedule IV
   a. The drug or other substance has a low potential for abuse relative to the drugs or other substances in schedule III.
   b. The drug or other substance currently has an accepted medical use in treatment in the United States.

    c. Abuse of the drug or other substance may lead to limited physical dependence or psychological dependence relative to the drugs or other substances in schedule III.

5. Schedule V

    a. The drug or other substance has a low potential for abuse relative to the drugs or other substances in schedule IV.

    b. The drug or other substance currently has an accepted medical use in treatment in the United States.

    c. Abuse of the drug or other substance may lead to limited physical dependence or psychological dependence relative to the drugs or other substances in schedule IV.

    d. A few select schedule V medications may be distributed to the patient without the need of a physician's prescription. In this instance, the patient and the pharmacist sign a log book entry that identifies the schedule V medication dispensed and the patient's identifying information, such as name and address.

ACTIVITY

Use the DEA website or another reference of choice to provide an example of two medications in each drug class. Provide the generic and a brand name for the medication:

1. Schedule I

2. Schedule II

3. Schedule III

4. Schedule IV

5. Schedule V

DEA SCHEDULED DRUG FORMS

DEA Form 222 is used to order C-I and C-II controlled substances from the distributor. The pharmacy technician may complete Form 222; however, the pharmacist must check over the form and sign the form before ordering the controlled substances.

The DEA is proposing to revise its regulations to provide an electronic equivalent to the DEA official order form. This revision will allow pharmacies to order schedule II substances electronically and maintain the records of these orders electronically. The proposed changes would reduce paperwork and transaction times. The changes will help to ensure the appropriate supply of controlled substances in the pharmacy.

DEA Form 41 is used in the event that controlled drugs must destroyed.

A detailed report of any theft or loss of controlled substances is completed using DEA Form 106.

ACTIVITY

Become familiar with DEA Forms 41 and 106.

1. Visit the U.S. Department of Justice DEA Office of Diversion Control website: *www.deadiversion.usdoj.gov*.
2. Scroll over *Reporting* on the left side of the screen.
3. Click on *Inventory of Drugs Surrendered* (DEA Form 41) and *Drug/Theft Loss* (DEA form 106).
4. Read through the directions for completing and submitting the forms.

QUESTIONS FOR REVIEW

Matching

Choose the item in column 2 that best matches each item in column 1.

1. Medications that are addictive and have a potential to be abused.	A. C-IV
	B. Chlorphentermine
2. Example of a C-II.	C. Morphine
3. Example of a C-III.	D. C-V
4. Has no accepted medicinal use.	E. DEA Form 222
5. Phenobarbital	F. Controlled drugs
6. May be distributed without a prescription.	G. C-I
7. Form used to order C-II medications.	

Short Answer

Write the word that best completes each statement.

Some schedule V medications may be distributed to a customer without a prescription provided that:

1. Distribution is made by a _____.
2. The purchaser is at least _____ years old.
3. The pharmacist knows the purchaser or requests _____.
4. A written record of distribution is kept. The record includes name and _____ of purchaser, name and _____ of controlled substance purchased, date of sale, and initials of pharmacist.
5. Limited _____ of C-V medications may be purchased within a 48-hour period.

Dr. Mark Paulsen   office: 800/777-2211
2100 Lake Avenue
Farmview, IA 51223

Patient Name__Cindy Klimer_____ **Date**__05/31/07_____

Address__129 Pear Dr. Okala, IA 51772_____

                                                                       Refill____7___Times

   Rx: Concerta 10mg po BID

      #60

Dr. Mark Paulsen

Product Selection Permitted   **Dispense As Written**

DEA NO._AP1234561_____

Address_____

1.   Is the prescription for Cindy Klimer valid? Why or why not?

Student Name _____ Date _____

Lab Partner _____

Grade/Comments _____

_____

Student Comments _____

_____

Brand-Generic

OBJECTIVES

- Point out the difference between the brand name, generic name, and chemical name of a drug.

- Classify common medication names in brand name or generic name category.

Pre-Lab Information

A drug reference book is a valuable tool for pharmacy technicians. For the drug reference book to be of value, it should be easy for you, the pharmacy technician, to use. It is essential that you become familiar with a drug reference book and use the book often so that you can obtain information in a quick, convenient fashion. In addition to a convenient design, your drug reference book of choice should contain current and concise information.

Suggested drug reference books:

Saunders Nursing Drug Handbook 2006
Mosby's Drug Guide for Nurses, sixth edition
Mosby's 2006 Drug Consult for Nurses

Review the suggested drug reference handbooks. While completing this lab, evaluate with which reference book you feel most comfortable.

BRAND/GENERIC NAMES

The name of a drug begins with a chemical name that describes its structure and components. Once the potential drug is under development, a generic name or nonproprietary name is assigned. When the drug is approved by the FDA, a brand name or proprietary name is introduced. Each drug will have only one generic name but may have many brand names.

Activity

1. List the brand and generic name of three medications in your pharmacy lab.
   a.
   b.
   c.

2. The following is a list of common drugs. Match the brand name of the drugs with the appropriate generic name by writing the letter of the correct answer on the line. Work with a partner to complete this activity.

Brand Names

1. ___ Cytoxan	21. ___ Lasix	41. ___ Intal
2. ___ Inderal	22. ___ Atrovent	42. ___ Cipro
3. ___ Keflex	23. ___ Benadryl	43. ___ Lotrimin
4. ___ Augmentin	24. ___ Ery-Tab	44. ___ Biaxin
5. ___ Foscavir	25. ___ Catapres	45. ___ Pepcid
6. ___ Coumadin	26. ___ Prozac	46. ___ Zoloft
7. ___ Levaquin	27. ___ Zyrtec	47. ___ Toradol
8. ___ Reglan	28. ___ Proventil	48. ___ Indocin
9. ___ Ativan	29. ___ Ceclor	49. ___ Hibiclens
10. ___ Zantac	30. ___ Procardia	50. ___ Zofran
11. ___ Tenormin	31. ___ Zovirax	
12. ___ Solu-Cortef	32. ___ Tegretol	
13. ___ Tylenol	33. ___ Dilantin	
14. ___ Amoxil	34. ___ Dilaudid	
15. ___ Diflucan	35. ___ Zithromax	
16. ___ Bactrim	36. ___ Oncovin	
17. ___ Minipress	37. ___ Lovenox	
18. ___ Decadron	38. ___ Celebrex	
19. ___ Valium	39. ___ Wellbutrin	
20. ___ Motrin	40. ___ Xanax	

Generic Names

a. amoxicillin
b. amoxicillin/potassium clavulanate
c. cefaclor
d. clarithromycin
e. sulfamethoxazole with trimethoprim
f. ciprofloxacin
g. erythromycin
h. cephalexin
i. levofloxacin
j. azithromycin
k. fluconazole
l. clotrimazole
m. chlorhexidine
n. foscarnet
o. acyclovir
p. cyclophosphamide

q. warfarin
r. enoxaparin
s. prazosin
t. propranolol
u. vincristine
v. atenolol
w. nifedipine
x. clonidine
y. metoclopramide
z. ondansetron
aa. famotidine
bb. ranitidine
cc. dexamethasone
dd. hydrocortisone
ee. acetaminophen
ff. hydromorphone
gg. phenytoin
hh. carbamazepine

ii. fluoxetine
jj. bupropion
kk. sertraline
ll. lorazepam
mm. diazepam
nn. alprazolam
oo. celecoxib
pp. indomethacin
qq. ibuprofen
rr. diphenhydramine
ss. ketorolac
tt. cetirizine
uu. cromolyn
vv. ipratropium
ww. albuterol
xx. furosemide

Student Name _____ Date _____

Lab Partner _____

Grade/Comments _____

_____

Student Comments _____

_____

Medication Errors

OBJECTIVE

• Obtain the skills necessary to report medication errors.

Pre-Lab Experience

Soundalike drugs have names that are spelled similarly even though they may be in a completely different class of medications. Soundalike and look-alike medications are potential causes of medication errors.

1. Access the ISMP List of Confused Drug Names: *www.ismp.org/tools/confuseddrugnames.pdf*.
2. Review the list of look-alike generic drug names.

REPORTING MEDICATION ERRORS

A medication error is any preventable event that may cause or lead to inappropriate medication use or patient harm while the medication is in the control of the health care professional, patient, or consumer. The responsibility of reporting medication errors should be shared between the pharmacy technician and the pharmacist as a standard of practice. Because pharmacy technicians are an integral part of filling a prescription, it is important for them to know the steps in reporting a medication error.

Errors may occur in a variety of forms:

1. Prescribing errors: problems with the prescription that require clarification with the prescriber before dispensing. This could involve poor handwriting and/or questions regarding dose and strength of prescribed medication.
2. During the process of selecting and filling a prescription an error may occur.

Methods of Reporting Medication Errors

1. FDA Form 3500 should be used for voluntary reporting.
2. The *MedWatch Online Voluntary Reporting Form* may be completed online by going to the MedWatch website: *www.fda.gov/medwatch.*
3. A medication error also may be reported by telephone. Make the report by calling MedWatch at 1-800-FDA-1088.

Activity

1. View the MedWatch Online Voluntary Reporting Form by accessing the MedWatch website: *www.fda.gov/safety/medwatch/howtoreport.*
   a. Click on *Reporting by Health Professions* listed below *Voluntary Reporting Using Form FDA 3500 for Consumers and Healthcare Professionals.*
   b. Become familiar with the information required on FDA Form 3500 for submission of medication error reporting.
2. Medication errors also may be reported to the Institute for Safe Medication Practices:
   a. Log onto *www.ismp.org.*
   b. Click on *Report Errors* at the top of the web page.
   c. Review information on ISMP Medication Errors Reporting Program (MERP).

QUESTIONS FOR REVIEW

1. True or false: MedWatch information given is meant to punish the pharmacy technician and to place blame on the pharmacist.
2. True or false: Medication errors may occur as a result of a stressful work environment.
3. List three look-alike generic medications, including the established name and the recommended name.

Student Name _____ Date _____

Lab Partner _____

Grade/Comments _____

_____

Student Comments _____

_____

Advanced Prescription Interpretation

OBJECTIVES

- Identify manufacturer's information on medication stock bottles.

- To gain increased awareness in prescription interpretation.

Pre-Lab Experience

Review error-prone abbreviations, symbols, and dose designations. A list can be obtained from the Institute for Safe Medication Practices at *www.ismp.org*.

ADVANCED PRESCRIPTION INTERPRETATION

Complete the prescription interpretation exercises:

- Write out all numbers.
- Be sure to use the appropriate verb.
- Write your answer in a complete sentence.

1. iii tsp MOM qd po

2. i gtts Timolol BID os

3. Norfloxacin tabs ii QID × 5d po

4. FESO4 324 mg po i qd

5. Omeprazole 20 mg cap ac po

6. 325 mg supp Tylenol PR PRN #5

7. MSO4 5 mg q 4h PRN pain IM

8. 50 mcg Nasonex spray ii sprays each nare qd

9. NTG 2% ung u.d. q 4-6h

10. ASA 650 mg BID

Student Name _____ Date _____

Lab Partner _____

Grade/Comments _____

_____

Student Comments _____

_____

Reference Materials

OBJECTIVE

- To become familiar with pharmacy-related reference materials.

Pre-Lab Information

Efficient use of any drug reference book requires an understanding of the organization and format of the book. Review the guidelines for use of each reference book before beginning the lab exercises. These guidelines can be found in the first few pages of the book near the introduction.

REFERENCE MATERIALS

Pharmacy technicians routinely use reference materials to obtain information on medication. In time, you will have a favorite reference source that is easy for you to use. Take this opportunity to explore various reference materials. Become familiar with the information found in each reference book.

Scenario: A local high school official visits the retail pharmacy where you are working. The high school official has three tablets in hand that were found in the high school locker room. Are you able to identify these tablets for the high school official? What reference resource would you use to make identification?

Drug Facts and Comparisons
- Contains information about prescription and over-the-counter (OTC) products
- Divides drugs into therapeutic or pharmacological groups, which allows for products that are most similar in content or use to be listed together
- Contains monographs detailing drug actions, indications, administration and dosage, adverse reactions, warnings, and more

Ident-A-Drug
- All pharmaceutical capsules or tablets are imprinted with identification codes. Ident-A-Drug reference allows you to identify any tablet or capsule by the code imprinted on it
- Includes NDC numbers, brand and generic names, manufacturers, and more

Physicians' Desk Reference (PDR)
- Information similar to manufacturer's drug package inserts
- Contains color-coded indexes arranged by brand and generic name of drug and an index arranged by drug category
- Product identification section
- *www.pdr.net*

Drug Topics Red Book
- Guide to average wholesale pricing (AWP)
- Product information on prescription drugs, OTC drugs, and reimbursable medical supplies
- Suggested retail prices for OTC products
- NDC numbers for all FDA-approved drugs
- Complete package information including dosage form, route of administration, strength, and size
- *Orange Book* codes: FDA Approved Drug Products with Therapeutic Equivalent Evaluations
- Vitamin comparison table: amounts of vitamins and minerals in more than 50 popular multivitamin products
- Common laboratory values
- Full color photos
- Guide to medicinal herbs

United States Pharmacopoeia Drug Information (USP DI)
- *www.usp.org*
- Published in two volumes. Volume 1 contains information for health care professionals, whereas volume 2 contains information for consumers.
- Recognized by the U.S. government as an approved source for off-label uses
- In depth information on prescription and OTC medications
- Contains drug monographs that provide information on drug interactions, side effects, dosing, and more

Drug Guide
- Drug information formatted into handbook
- Includes pregnancy category

- Drug classifications, actions and therapeutic effects, uses and unlabeled uses
- Route and dosage
- Drug guide handbooks available that specialize in intravenous medications

Student Directions

Drug information is readily available on the Internet; however, for the following lab exercises, you are instructed to make use of the bound or printed edition of each resource. Referencing the bound edition allows for practice in obtaining accurate information in an efficient manner.

1. Using *Drug Facts and Comparisons,* find the following information:
   Helpful Hint: Look up individual drugs by using the index in the back of the book. Find drug classes by using the table of contents at the front of the book.

   a. What drug groups or subgroups are listed in the Gastrointestinal Agents chapter? List three.

   b. In what dosage form is guaifenesin available?

   c. What medication has the same active ingredient(s) as amiodarone HCl?

   d. What is an OTC sugar-free alternative to calcium carbonate?

   e. What company distributes Neoral?

   f. What is the product identification for Neoral soft gelatin capsule?

2. Using *Ident-A-Drug,* find the following information:
   Helpful Hint: Look up the number or letter that is farthest to the left of the tablet. Entries are listed in the *Ident-A-Drug* reference book in alphabetical and numerical order.

   a. The round tablet is green with black print. One side of the tablet bears the markings 67. The other side of the tablet bears the markings SL. What is the brand name of this medication? Into what drug class does the medication fall?

b. The capsule is blue and white with black print. One side of the tablet is marked with Z4804. What is the generic name and strength of this medication?

3. Using the *PDR*, find the following information:
   Helpful Hint: When looking up product information for a drug, first look in the manufacturer's index to find out who manufacturers the product and the page number of the product.
   a. Identify the product with the markings of 10 on one side and OC on the opposite side.

   b. Who is the manufacturer of Tamiflu? For what is Tamiflu indicated?

4. Using the *Drug Topics Red Book*, find the following information:
   Helpful Hint: The Product Listings section of the *Drug Topics Red Book* is perused with tables that indicate route of administration symbols, *Orange Book* codes, standard dosage form abbreviations, and many others.
   a. List five drugs that should never be crushed.

   b. What is the look-alike, soundalike drug for Humulin?

   c. What is the route of administration for Eryzole? What is the *Orange Book* code for Eryzole? What is AWP for Eryzole 100 mL? What does *PDR* represent as listed under Eryzole?

5. Using *USP DI* find the following information:
   Helpful Hint: Drug classes are arranged alphabetically. If the drug class is unknown, look up the drug name by using the general index at the back of the book.
   a. What drug category is Parnate?

   b. What may be a more frequent side/adverse effect with the use of Parnate?

   c. List two precautions the patient should take while using Parnate.

6. Using a drug guide reference book find the following information:
   Helpful Hint: Use the index in the back of the book to look up drugs by
brand or generic name.
   a. What is the pregnancy category for Namenda? For Pontocaine?

   b. According to the FDA Pregnancy Category appendix in the drug
      guide, which category signifies a medication to be contraindicated
      during pregnancy? Which category signifies positive evidence of
      human fetal risk?

   c. What is the availability of caffeine?

   Intravenous Medications Drug Guide Handbook
   d. What are the compatibility requirements of azithromycin?

Student Name _____ Date _____

Lab Partner _____

Grade/Comments _____

_____

Student Comments _____

_____

Conversions

OBJECTIVE

- Become comfortable with basic mathematical operations involved in pharmacy technician math.

Pre-Lab Experience

You may desire a refresher course on basic mathematical operations. Visit *www.math.com* for review activities in addition, subtraction, multiplication, division, fraction/decimal conversion, and metric conversion.

CONVERSIONS

Essential to the proper handling of drugs and the preparation of prescriptions is understanding mathematical operations. A pharmacy technician should know measurement units, number systems, and mathematical operations.

Exercises

Complete the following exercises. Show all of your work in calculating the answer.

1. Convert the following fractions to percents:
    a. 60/100 _____
    b. 80/100 _____
    c. 12/100 _____

2. Convert the following percents to decimals:
    a. 50% _____
    b. 12.5% _____
    c. 99% _____

3. Convert the following:
    a. 500 g = _____ mg
    b. 10 kg = _____ g
    c. 250 mL = _____ L
    d. 325 mg = _____ g
    e. 102 kg = _____ lb

4. Calculate the following:
    a. 1/2 + 5/6 = _____
    b. 3/8 − 1/16 = _____
    c. 0.75 × 1.2 = _____

5. Write the following Roman numerals as Arabic numerals:
    a. VII _____
    b. XCII _____
    c. CCVII _____

6. Write the following Arabic numerals as Roman numerals:
    a. 27 _____
    b. 94 _____

7. How many pounds do the following patients weigh?
    a. 14 kg = _____ lb
    b. 106 kg = _____ lb

8. Convert the following amounts:
    a. 8 fl oz = _____ mL
    b. 4 tsp = _____ mL
    c. 11 oz = _____ g

Student Name _____ Date _____

Lab Partner _____

Grade/Comments _____

_____

Student Comments _____

_____

Pharmacy Office

Reports: Inventory Management

OBJECTIVES

- Become familiar with pharmacy reports generated through pharmacy-specific computer software.

- Gain a base understanding of the concept of inventory.

Pre-Lab Information

An inventory is a listing of goods or items that a pharmacy will use in its operation. A pharmacy develops an inventory based on what medications the pharmacist expects to need. The goal of inventory management is to have drugs available when they are needed. Because inventory management is a job responsibility of the technician, you must be familiar with the inventory system used in your practice setting.

INVENTORY MANAGEMENT/REPORTING

1. Place the *Visual SuperScript* CD into your computer. Enter your password.
2. Click on *Data* on the menu toolbar located on the top of the screen.
3. Click on *Drugs* from the Data submenu.
4. Click the green *Drug and Packaging* tab.

5. Review options on this screen/form by reading the screen tips. This is done by slowly guiding the mouse pointer to each text box or field. Leave the pointer on the field until the screen tip appears.
6. Click on the *Add Drug by NDC* tab located at the top left of the form.
7. Type in the NDC for Flomax: 00597-0058-01.
8. Add the drug to the pharmacy inventory by clicking on the *Add Drug* tab.
9. Exit from the *Drug* screen/form by clicking the red X in the upper right corner.
10. Click on *Reports* on the menu toolbar located on the top of the screen.
11. Move the mouse pointer over *Daily Prescription Log* and then click on *Daily Rx Log.*
12. A *Daily Rx Log* submenu appears. Type the following dates in the *Include Records From* text boxes: 07/02/2002 to today's date.
13. Click on the *Preview* tab.
14. A record of dispensed prescriptions is generated according to the dispensed dates indicated on the *Daily Rx Log.*
15. Exit the dispensed prescription form by clicking the black X in the upper right corner of the screen.
16. Investigate other reports available for use on the *Visual SuperScript* pharmacy software.
17. Answer the questions.

Note: Software is not included with this manual.

INVENTORY MANAGEMENT/PURCHASE ORDER

1. What company manufacturers Flomax?
2. What is the package size of Flomax?
3. What dispensed medications are listed on the computer-generated form from the *Daily Rx* menu?

Student Name _____ Date _____

Lab Partner _____

Grade/Comments _____

_____

Student Comments _____

_____

Business Math

OBJECTIVES

- Calculate pharmacy business problems: inventory turnover, markup, and profit.

- Demonstrate temperature and prescription conversions.

Pre-Lab Information

Pharmacy technicians use basic math skills every day while in the career field. Understanding math calculations, conversions, and measurements is essential. In addition to calculations involving patient care, pharmacy technicians work with calculations on the business management side of pharmacy. The business calculations involve accounting practices such as inventory, accounts receivable, and accounts payable.

AWP: average wholesale price
AMP: average manufacturer's price
Overhead: general cost of doing business
Capitation fee: form of reimbursement by the insurance company in which the pharmacy is paid a set monthly fee
Inventory: all items that are available for resale in the pharmacy business
Days' supply: average length of time items are in inventory, that is, how many days a business could continue selling using only its existing inventory; 25 to 30 days is common goal for days' supply
Turnover rate: the number of times goods within pharmacy inventory are sold during the year

CONVERSIONS: PART II

Complete the following exercises. Show all of your work.
Convert the following measurements:

1. 77 mg = _____ gr
2. 1/4 gr = _____ mg
3. 6 oz = _____ mL
4. 80 mL = _____ oz
5. 70 kg = _____ g
6. 25 L = _____ mL

Perform the necessary mathematical operations for the following selling price problems:

1. $9.07 with a markup of 27%
2. What is the percent of profit made on a product that cost the pharmacy $30.00 and will be sold for $34.00?
3. A pharmacy has an inventory of $270,400. Last week the total sales were $32,980 and the profit was $5,798. What is the pharmacy's days' supply? If the inventory goal is 30 days, was the goal reached?

Temperature Conversions

$$C = 5/9(F - 32) \qquad F = 32 + 9/5C$$

- $C = 5/9(F - 32)$ or subtract 32 and divide by 1.8 to obtain C
- $F = 32 + 9/5C$ or multiply by 1.8 and add 32 to obtain F

Student Note: Use the formula that you are most comfortable with.

1. 212 F = _____ C
2. 98 C = _____ F

Prescription Conversions

1. You receive an order to compound #24, 250-mg capsules. How many 1.5-g tablets must be crushed to obtain enough drug to compound this order?
2. You receive a prescription for i 250 mg tab PO TID × 10 d. The pharmacy carries 500-mg tablets of this medicine. How many 500-mg tablets are needed to fill the order?

Student Name _____ Date _____

Lab Partner _____

Grade/Comments _____

_____

Student Comments _____

_____

Prior Authorizations

OBJECTIVE

- Indicate the procedure for securing prior authorizations for medications.

Pre-Lab Information

PA: prior authorization

The purpose of drug prior authorization is to promote proper use of medications, thereby effectively managing associated costs.

When a prior authorization is submitted, insurance companies will evaluate whether there are other less expensive medications that may be an option for the patient. Reviewers evaluate the clinical information obtained from the Prior Authorization Request Form.

Formulary: A drug formulary is a listing of prescription medicines that are covered by the insurance provider for reimbursement. The key difference between an *open* and a *closed formulary* is that specific drugs on the *closed formulary* may be reimbursed only if medical exception or prior authorization is obtained.

PRIOR AUTHORIZATIONS

Insurers sometimes reject a prescription claim that is submitted for reimbursement. There are a number of reasons for rejections. The pharmacy team must resolve the problem. Most of the insurance billing or adjudication problems can be solved by talking with an insurance representative on the telephone and/or by discussing the rejection with the patient.

Certain medications require prior authorization to ensure that a drug is medically necessary and part of a specific treatment plan. Prior authorization program guidelines may consist of the following:

- The prescribing physician should notify the insurance carrier in advance about the medical condition that requires the use of drugs that appear on the prior authorization list; getting the authorization in advance will prevent delays at the pharmacy.
- Once the drug is authorized, the prescription can be filled at any participating pharmacy.
- For most drugs, the authorization is valid for 1 year.

Following is a list of medications that may require prior authorization:

PRESCRIPTION NAME

AcipHex (effective 05/01/2004)*

Arava†

Celebrex (effective 08/15/2003)

Cialis (has quantity limit of six tablets per 30 days)

Desoxyn

Dexedrine

Levitra (has quantity limit of six tablets per 30 days)

Mobic (effective 03/01/2005)

Nexium (effective 05/01/2004)*

Omeprazole (effective 05/01/2004)*

Oral contraceptives (if your plan does not cover this benefit)

Prevacid (effective 05/01/2004)*

Prevacid NapraPAC (effective 05/01/2004)*

Prilosec (effective 05/01/2004)*

Progesterone (compounded forms)

Protonix (effective 05/01/2004)*

Provigil (effective 03/01/2005)

Sporanox

Topical tretinoin (Retin-A and Avita; if you are over 35 years of age)

Vfend

Viagra† (has quantity limit of six tablets per 30 days)

Wellbutrin SR

Wellbutrin XL

Zegerid (effective 09/13/2004)*

*Prior authorization required after 90-day total supply filled in a rolling calendar year.
†Approval remains in effect as long as your coverage remains the same.

ACTIVITY

1. When would a prior authorization be needed?

2. Fill out a prior authorization request for the patient Samantha Jones. What should you tell Samantha after she requests the refill and the insurance now is requiring a prior authorization?

3. With a partner, role-play a phone call to a Dr. Mark Paulsen's office for a prior authorization request for your pharmacy patient, Samantha Jones.

4. What are some tips for handling a prior authorization request?

Patient Samantha Jones

Patient Samantha Jones (DOB 01/15/1979) stops in GetWell Pharmacy with a prescription for Nexium. She has been taking Zantac and famotidine for the past 6 months with no relief from stomach pains. Ms. Jone's insurance company is requiring a prior authorization before paying for the Nexium.

Dr. Mark Paulsen   office: 800/777-2211
2100 Lake Avenue
Farmview, IA 51223

Patient Name __Samantha Jones_____ Date__6/20/07_____

  Address_____

        Refill_____1____Times
        Rx: Nexium 20mg
               i po qd
               take 1 hour a meals

Dr. Mark Paulsen

Product Selection Permitted   **Dispense As Written**

DEA NO._____

Address_____

GENERAL PRIOR AUTHORIZATION REQUEST FORM

Fax Completed Information to 999/444-1112

Patient Information

Last Name_____ First Name_____ MI_____

Patient

ID_____ DOB_____ Sex_____

First date of service _____ Last date of service _____

Diagnosis_____

Medication Information

Strength_____ Quantity per Month_____ Length of Therapy_____

Medication Currently Taking_____

Directions on Current

Medication_____

Medication to Prior

Authorize_____

Please list medications patient has tried for this diagnosis.

Medication Name	Dosage	Date(s) of Therapy	Outcome

EXPLANATION OF NECESSITY FOR PROCEDURES (Attach supporting x-ray films, lab reports, operative reports, and discharge summaries if indicated.)

PROVIDER INFORMATION

Medical Assistance Provider Number

_____

I certify that the information given in this form is a true and accurate medical indication for the procedures required. All other treatment to correct this problem has been exhausted.

_____

_____

Provider Signature/Date

Provider Name: _____

Address: _____

_____

Provider Phone # _____ Fax #_____

E-Mail _____

Student Name _____ Date _____

Lab Partner _____

Grade/Comments _____

_____

Student Comments _____

_____

Medicare

OBJECTIVE

- Gain an understanding of Medicare Prescription Drug Insurance.

Pre-Lab Experience

Centers for Medicare and Medicare Services provide an online handbook available to learn more about Medicare insurance. Topics covered in the handbook, *Medicare and You*, include costs, coverage and drug plans.

Access Medicare information at *www.medicare.gov*. Click on *Medicare and You 2011 Handbook*.

UNDERSTANDING MEDICARE PRESCRIPTION PLANS

It is important for the pharmacy technician to have a basic understanding of prescription drug coverage. This lab focuses on Medicare Part D Prescription Drug Benefits.

Medicare is insurance provided by the government to citizens 65 years or older and a group of citizens who are disabled. Eighty-five percent of the population in the United States is eligible for Medicare. This means that as a pharmacy technician you will provide service to a large percentage of patients who are enrolled in a Medicare prescription drug plan. Medicare has different coverage types: Part A pays for inpatient hospital, skilled nursing facility, and some home health care; Part B helps cover doctors' services, outpatient hospital care, medically necessary supplies, and some other medical services that Medicare Part A does not cover; and Part D went into effect on January 1, 2006. Before the rollout of Part D, Medicare Health Insurance did not cover prescription medication costs for senior citizens.

Basically, individuals who are enrolled in Medicare Part D pay a part of the cost of their brand-name or generic prescription medication. Enrollees also pay a co-payment when their prescription medication is purchased. The amount of co-payment that is due at purchase, and the percentage that Medicare Part D will pay for the prescription medication varies depending on the insurance plan in which the patient is enrolled. On the average, individual states offer 40 different prescription drug plans to Medicare enrollees.

1. Log onto *www.medicare.gov/find-a-plan*.
2. Enter your zip code to bring up Medicare Prescription Drug Plans offered in your state.
3. You may also choose the option to find and compare Medigap Policies in your state.
4. Answer the following questions:
   a. Which drug plan in your state offers the lowest premium?

   b. What is the organization that offers the prescription drug plan with the lowest premium?

   c. How many top 100 drugs are included in the formulary of this prescription drug plan?

   d. What is the deductible for drugs in this prescription drug plan?

Student Name _____ Date _____

Lab Partner _____

Grade/Comments _____

_____

Student Comments _____

_____

Bibliography

WEBSITES

Some information used in this textbook was obtained from the following websites:

1. American Society of Health-System Pharmacists. www.ashp.org.
2. Bronx Medical Malpractice/SWI Digital, Inc. www.bronxmedicalmalpractice.com.
3. Containment Technologies Group, Inc., Mobile Isolation Chambers. www.mic4.com/products/.
4. Department of Health and Human Services Center for Disease Control. www.cdc.gov.
5. Lasco Services. www.lascoservices.com.
6. Management Sciences for Health: The Provider's Guide to Quality and Culture. http://erc.msh.org.
7. McKesson Corporation. www.mckesson.com.
8. National Cleanrooms. http://n-p.com/cleanrooms/practice.asp.
9. Professional Compounding Centers of America. www.pccarx.com.
10. RX Insider. www.rxinsider.com.
11. South Dakota Department of Social Services. http://dss.sd.gov/.
12. The Henry J. Kaiser Family Foundation. www.kff.org.
13. The Manager's Electronic Resource Center. http://erc.msh.org/.
14. The Med Supply Guide. www.themedsupplyguide.com.
15. The National Healthcare Providers Service Organization. www.npso.com.
16. United States Department of Health and Human Services. www.hhs.gov.
17. United States Drug Enforcement Administration. www.dea.gov.
18. Venture Line. www.ventureline.com.

PUBLICATIONS

Ballington D: *Pharmacy practice for technicians*, ed 2, St. Paul, Minn., 2006, EMC Paradigm.

Ballington D, Green T: *Pharmacy calculations for technicians*, ed 3, St. Paul, Minn., 2006, EMC Paradigm.

Buchanan E, Schneider P: *Compounding sterile preparations*, ed 2, Bethesda, Maryland, 2005, American Society of Health-System Pharmacists.

Crane A: *Rx success: compounding techniques and theory for the pharmacy technician*, Menomonee Falls, Wisconsin, 2002, Salt and Light Enterprises, LLC.

Laska L. "Overworked and Error-Prone Pharmacist Misfills Prescription: Confidential Settlement." *Medical Malpractice Verdicts, Settlements & Experts*, 17, no. 10 (October 2001): 49.

Mosby's medical, nursing, and allied health dictionary: St. Louis, 2006, Elsevier.

VIDEO

Power L, Jorgenson J: *Safe handling of hazardous drugs: video training program*, Bethesda, Maryland, 2006, American Society of Health-System Pharmacists.

Index

A

Accelerated approval, Food and Drug Administration approval process and, 154
Acetaminophen, 165
Acetylsalicylic acid, 170
AcipHex, 186
Acquired immunodeficiency syndrome, approval of drugs for, 155
Active ingredient, over-the-counter labeling and, 146
Acyclovir, 165
ADDD. *See* Automated drug dispensing system
Advisory committee, Food and Drug Administration approval process and, 153
Africans, cultural competence and, 131
AIDS. *See* Acquired immunodeficiency syndrome
Air bubble, removal of, from syringe, 99, 102
Airborne contamination, 84
Albuterol, 165
Alcohol
    aseptic technique and, 88
    sterilization of vial with, 98
Allegra, 38
Allergy, patient, medication order and, 56
Alprazolam, 165
Alternative remedies, 130
American Diabetes Association, website of, 34
American Indians, cultural competence and, 131
Amiodarone HCl, 173
Amoxicillin, 165
Amoxicillin/potassium clavulanate, 165
Amoxil, 164
AMP. *See* Average manufacturer's price
Ampule
    aseptic compounding and, 82
    withdrawing liquid from, 101-104
Animal testing, drug approval process and, 150, 157
Anteroom, definition of, 87
Antibiotics, 81
    intravenous, preparation of, 101
"Approvable" designation, Food and Drug Administration approval process and, 154-155, 157
Arab people, cultural competence and, 132
Arabic numerals, conversion of, 177
Arava, 186
ASA. *See* Acetylsalicylic acid
Aseptic IV compounding pharmacy, 81-83
Aseptic technique, 81-115
    checklist for, 86
    description of, 85
    gowning and, 87-89
    hand washing and, 85-86
    sterile compounding and, 94
Asians, cultural competence and, 131
Aspirin, 170
Atenolol, 165
Ativan, 164
Atrovent, 164

Attitude, communication skills and, 122
Augmentin, 164
Automated compounding system, aseptic compounding and, 82
Automated drug dispensing system, 37-40
Automated prescription system, 61
Automation, pharmacy, 60-61
Auxiliary label, 3, 4
    intravenous bag labeling with, 108
Avapro, lawsuit involving, 138
Avara, lawsuit involving, 138
Average manufacturer's price, 183
Average wholesale price, 183
Avita, 186
AWP. *See* Average wholesale price
Azithromycin, 165, 175
AZT. *See* Zidovudine

B

Bactrim, 164
Baker Cassette, 38
Baker cell, 37-40
Balance, use of, 65-67
Bar coding, 61
Barrel, syringe, 98
Becton/Dickinson, website of, 97
Behavior, standards of, 136
Benadryl, 164
Bevel, syringe, 98
Biaxin, 164
Billing information, consumers' rights and, 44
Biological license application, 156
Biological safety cabinet, 96-96
BLA. *See* Biological license application
Blood glucose
    monitoring of, 34-36
    normal level of, 35
Blood testing, procedure for, 35
Body language, 119
BSC. *See* Biological safety cabinet
Bupropion, 165
Business math, 183-184

C

Caffeine, 175
Calcium carbonate, 173
Cancer, approval of drugs for, 155
Cane, fitting patient for, 31
Capacity, conversion table for, 148
Capitation fee, definition of, 183
Carbamazepine, 165
Cardiovascular disease, approval of drugs for, 155
Catapres, 164
CBER. *See* Center for Biologics Evaluation and Research
CDER. *See* Center for Drug Evaluation and Research
Ceclor, 164
Cefaclor, 165
Celebrex, 164, 186

Celecoxib, 165
Center for Biologics Evaluation and Research, 156
Center for Drug Evaluation and Research, 152, 153, 154, 155, 156, 157
    website of, 149, 166
Centigrade temperature, conversion of, 184
Cephalexin, 38, 165
Certificate of medical necessity, home medical equipment and, 31
Cetaphil, 71, 72
Cetirizine, 165
Charge log
    example of, 50
    in mail order pharmacy, 47
Checking area, in mail order pharmacy, 47
Chemical name, 163, 164
Chlorhexidine, 165
Chlorpheniramine maleate, 147
Chlorphentermine, 161
Chronic myeloid leukemia, approval of drugs for, 154
Cialis, 186
Cipro, 164
Ciprofloxacin, 165
Claim, rejection of, 15
Clarithromycin, 165
Class A prescription balance, 66-67
Class action lawsuit, example of, 137
Clean room, 84
Clicking, definition of, 16
Clinical data, drug approval process and, 156-157
Clinical trials
    drug approval process and, 151, 152, 157
    size of, 153
Clonidine, 165
Closed formulary, definition of, 185
Clotrimazole, 165
CML. See Chronic myeloid leukemia
Coat, aseptic technique and, 88
Code of Ethics for Pharmacy Technicians, 135-136
Common phrases, Spanish translation of, 128-129
Communication, 119-126
    effect of culture on, 129-132
    nonverbal, 119-120, 131
    stereotyping and, 124-126
    on telephone, 121-122
Competence, code of ethics and, 136
Compounded sterile preparation, 84
Compounding
    basic equipment for, 68-69
    definition of, 68
    exercises for, 71-74, 75-78
    extemporaneous, 65-78
    horizontal laminar airflow hood and, 93-94
    medication in intravenous bag and, 109-110
    sterile, 94
Compression stockings, 32-33
Consumers' rights, 42
Contamination
    airborne, 84
    gowning and, 87
    minimization of, 85
    prevention of, 94
Controlled drugs, 22, 158-162
    DEA Form 222 for, 160
Controlled trials, drug approval process and, 151
Conversion tables, 147-148, 176-177
Conversions, 184
Coumadin, 164
Counseling, communication skills and, 123
Counting tray, cleaning of, 7, 8
Critical area, definition of, 93
Cromolyn, 165
CSP. See Compounded sterile preparation

Cultural competence, 131-132
Culture
    communication and, 129-132
    language and, 130
Culture Quiz, 129-132
Cyclophosphamide, 165
Cytoxan, 164

D

Data entry
    in mail order pharmacy, 46-47
    for prescription, 17-18
    for prescription refill, 27-29
Date of birth, inpatient prescription processing and, 55
DAW. See Dispense as written
Days' supply, definition of, 183
De-gowning, aseptic technique and, 88
DEA. See Drug Enforcement Administration
Decadron, 164
Decimals, conversion of, 177
Degloving, aseptic technique and, 88
Dependency, scheduled drugs and, 159, 160
Desoxyn, 186
Dexamethasone, 165
Dexedrine, 186
Diabetes, management of, 34-35
Diagnosis, patient, medication order and, 56
Diazepam, 165
Diet, cultural competence and, 130, 132
Diflucan, 164
Dilantin, 164
Dilaudid, 164
Diluent, reconstituting powder and, 106, 107
Diphenhydramine, 165
Disinfectant, aseptic technique and, 88
Disinfectant solution, 8
Dispense as written, 18
Dispensing, in mail order pharmacy, 47
Dispensing system, 61
Division of Scientific Investigations, 156
DME. See Durable medical equipment
DOB. See Date of birth
Dosages, over-the-counter labeling and, 146
Dosing, pediatric, compounded medication for, 75
Drams, conversion factors for, 147, 148
Drive-thru window, 127
Drops, conversion factors for, 148
Drug design, 149-157
Drug Enforcement Administration, 158
Drug Enforcement Agency
    Form 41 from, 161
    Form 106 from, 161
    Form 222 from, 160
Drug Facts and Comparisons, 172, 173
Drug Guide, 172-173
Drug reference book, 163
Drug Topics Red Book, 172, 174
Drugs
    approval process for, Food and Drug Administration and, 149-150
    brand names of, 163-165
    chemical names of, 163
    controlled, 22, 158-162
    effectiveness of, drug approval process and, 155
    generic names of, 163-165
    hazardous, 112-115
    Schedule I, 159
    Schedule II, 159
    Schedule III, 159
    Schedule IV, 159-160
    scheduled, 158-162
Dry powder, reconstitution of, 105-106

DSI. *See* Division of Scientific Investigations
Durable medical equipment, 30-33

E

Eastern Europeans, cultural competence and, 131
Edit box, definition of, 16
Electronic balance, 65
Eli Lilly and Company, lawsuit involving, 136-137
Enoxaparin, 165
Ery-Tab, 164
Erythromycin, 165
Eryzole, 174
Ethics, 135-139
Ethyl alcohol, cleaning with, 91
ETOH. *See* Ethyl alcohol
Expiration date, intravenous bag labeling with, 108

F

Fahrenheit temperature, conversion of, 184
Famotidine, 165
Fax form, example of, 26
FDA. *See* Food and Drug Administration
Federal Food, Drug, and Cosmetic Act, 159
Ferrous sulfate, 170
FESO4. *See* Ferrous sulfate
Flomax, 182
Flow hood, aseptic technique and, 85
Fluconazole, 165
Fluid drams, conversion factors for, 148
Fluid ounces, conversion factors for, 148
Fluoxetine, 165
Folk remedies, 130
Food and Drug Administration, 149
    Form 3500 from, medication error reported on, 167
    list of scheduled drugs from, 158
    review process of, 150-157
Formulary, definition of, 185
Foscarnet, 165
Foscavir, 164
Fractions, conversion of, 176
Function key, definition of, 16
Furosemide, 165

G

Gallipot, website of, 75
Gallon, conversion factors for, 148
Garb
    aseptic compounding and, 82
    cleanroom, 87
    definition of, 87
Geometric dilution, 72
Gleevec, 154
Gloves
    aseptic technique and, 87, 88
    hazardous drug handling and, 113
Glucose monitor, 34-36
Gowning
    aseptic technique and, 87-89
    technique for, 89
Gowning up, aseptic technique and, 85
Graduated cylinder, compounding and, 68
Grains, conversion factors for, 147
Grams, conversion factors for, 147
Guaifenesin, 173

H

Hair cover, aseptic technique and, 87
Half-life, nuclear pharmacy preparations and, 113
Hand hygiene, 5-6
Hand washing, 5-6
    aseptic technique and, 85-86
    checklist for, 86

Hazardous drugs, 112-115
Health information
    consumers' rights regarding, 42, 44
    privacy rights and, 43-45
Health Insurance Portability and Accountability Act, 20, 25, 28, 41-45
    pharmacy drive-thru window and, 127
    website for information on, 43, 44, 45
Healthcare Providers Service Organization, website of, 139
Height, patient, medication order and, 56
HEPA. *See* High-efficiency particulate air filter
Hibiclens, 164
High-efficiency particulate air filter, 90, 91, 93
Hinduism, cultural competence and, 132
HIPAA. *See* Health Insurance Portability and Accountability Act
HIV. *See* Human immunodeficiency virus
HME. *See* Home medical equipment
Home care organization, 105
Home medical equipment, 30-33
Horizontal flow hood, aseptic technique and, 85
Horizontal laminar airflow hood
    cleaning of, 90-94
    compounding and, 93-94
Hormone replacement therapy, compounded medication for, 75
Hospital room number, patient, medication order and, 56
Household measures, conversion table for, 148
Hub, syringe, 98
Human immunodeficiency virus, approval of drugs for, 154
Human testing, drug approval process and, 150
Humulin, 174
Hydrocodone, 38
Hydrocortisone, 165
Hydromorphone, 165
Hygiene, hand, 5-6

I

Ibuprofen, 165
Icon, definition of, 16
Ident-A-Drug, 172, 173
Identification, patient, medication order and, 56
Illness, belief system and, 130
Imatinib mesylate, 154
Inactive ingredients, over-the-counter labeling and, 146
IND. *See* Investigational new drug application
Inderal, 164
Indocin, 164
Indomethacin, 165
Infection
    hand washing for prevention of, 5
    life-threatening, approval of drugs for, 155
Infusion clinic, 105
Ingredients, intravenous bag labeling with, 108
Injection port, 110
Institute for Safe Medication Practices, 55
    website of, 55, 169
Institutional review board, 151
Insurance
    home medical equipment and, 31
    information for, 14
Insurance card, 12-15
Insurance claim
    for home medical equipment, 30, 31
    rejection of, 15
Insurance company, prior authorization required by, 185
Intal, 164
International Standards Organization, 84
Internet pharmacy, patient protection and, 137-138
Interpreter, medical information through, 129, 130
Intravenous bag, introducing liquid into, 108-111
Intravenous medication, preparation of, 101
Intravenous Medications Drug Guide Handbook, 175
Intravenous piggyback, 102
Inventory, definition of, 183

Inventory management, 181-182
Investigational new drug application, 151, 157
Invoice
    example of, 48
    mail order pharmacy and, 47
Ipratropium, 165
IRB. *See* Institutional review board
Islam, cultural competence and, 132
ISO. *See* International Standards Organization
Isopropyl alcohol, 7
    aseptic technique and, 88

K

Keflex, 164
Ketorolac, 165
Kilogram, conversion factors for, 147

L

Label printing software, 61
Labeling
    over-the-counter, 145-148
    of scheduled drugs, 159
LAFW. *See* Laminar airflow workbench
Laminar airflow hood
    aseptic compounding and, 82
    horizontal, cleaning of, 90-94
    vertical, cleaning of, 95-96
Laminar airflow workbench
    aseptic compounding and, 82
    cleaning of, 90-94
Language, culture and, 130
Lasix, 164
Latin Americans, cultural competence and, 131
Law, pharmacy, 140-142
Lawsuit, example of, 136-137
Leukemia, chronic myeloid, approval of drugs for, 154
Levaquin, 164
Levitra, 186
Levofloxacin, 165
Liability insurance, 139
Lip, syringe, 98
Listening skills, 119
Lollipop mold, 75
Lorazepam, 165
Lotrimin, 164
Lovenox, 164
Luer-Lok syringe, 82

M

Mail log
    example of, 51
    in mail order pharmacy, 47
Mail order prescription, 46-52
Mail room, 46
Manufacturer, drug approval process and, 155, 157
Mask, aseptic technique and, 87, 88
Master formula sheet, 69, 76
    example of, 70, 73
Material safety data sheet, 112
Mathematics, business, 183-184
McKesson, website of, 60
Medical equipment, home, 30-33
Medicare, 190-191
    home medical equipment and, 31
Medicare Part D Prescription Drug Benefits, 190-191
Medication
    approval of, by Food and Drug Administration, 149
    brand names of, 163-165
    C-I, 160
    C-II, 160, 161
    C-III, 161
    C-IV, 161

Medication—cont'd
    compounded, 75
    controlled, 22
    errors in, 166-168
        reduction of, 60
    generic names of, 163-165
    hazardous, 112-115
    intravenous, preparation of, 101
    intravenous bag for, 109-110
    labeling of, 145
    oral, counting of, 7-8
    over-the-counter
        consumer information on label of, 149
        labeling of, 145
    powdered, 106
    withdrawing of
        from ampule, 101-104
        from vial, 97-100
Medication order, 56-58
    example of, 56-58
Medicine, belief system and, 130
MedWatch, website of, 167
MedWatch Online Voluntary Reporting Form, 167
Merck Research Laboratories, 152
Methylcellulose, 75
Metoclopramide, 165
Milligrams, conversion factors for, 147
Milliliters, conversion factors for, 148
Minims, conversion factors for, 148
Minipress, 164
Minitroche mold, 75
Mixing, reconstitution of powder and, 107
Mobic, 186
Mobility equipment, 31
Montelukast sodium, 152
Morphine, 161
Morphine sulfate, 170
Mortar, compounding and, 68, 76
Mosby's 2006 Drug Consult for Nurses, 163
Mosby's Drug Guide for Nurses, 163
Motrin, 164
MSDS. *See* Material safety data sheet
MSO4. *See* Morphine sulfate
Muslims, cultural competence and, 132

N

NABP. *See* National Association of Boards of Pharmacy
Name, patient, medication order and, 56
Namenda, 175
Narcotics, 158-162
    schedule II, prescription filling for, 158
Nasonex, 170
National Association of Boards of Pharmacy, 141
Native Americans, cultural competence and, 131
NDA. *See* New drug application
Needle
    aseptic compounding and, 82
    parts of, 97
    withdrawing liquid from ampule with, 102-103
Neoral, 173
New drug application, drug approval process and, 151-152, 157
New molecular entity, drug approval process and, 156
Nexium, 186
NIDPOE. *See* Notice of Initiation of Disqualification
    Proceedings and Opportunities to Explain
Nifedipine, 165
Nitroglycerine, 170
NME. *See* New molecular entity
Nonverbal communication, 119-120, 131
Norfloxacin, 170
"Not approvable" designation, Food and Drug Administration
    approval process and, 154-155, 157

Notice of Initiation of Disqualification Proceedings and Opportunities to Explain, 156
NTG. *See* Nitroglycerine
Nuclear pharmacy, 113

O

Office of Diversion and Control, 161
Omeprazole, 170, 186
Oncovin, 164
Ondansetron, 165
Open formulary, definition of, 185
Oral contraceptives, 186
Oral medication, counting of, 7-8
Order entry, in mail order pharmacy, 47
OTC. *See* Over-the-counter medication
OTC Drug Facts Label, 145
Ounces, conversion factors for, 147
Over-the-counter medication, 19
    labeling for, 145-148
Overhead, definition of, 183

P

PA. *See* Prior authorization
Packaging, thermal medication, 61
Parchment paper, compounding and, 69, 72
Parenteral bag, aseptic compounding and, 82
Parke-Davis History of Pharmacy in Pictures, website of, 81
Parnate, 174
Particulate, definition of, 90
Patient identification, intravenous bag labeling with, 108
Patient information
    medication order and, 55, 56
    for retail prescription, 19-20
    Spanish phrases for, 128-129
Patient name, intravenous bag labeling with, 108
PCCA. *See* Professional Compounding Centers of America
PDR. *See* Physicians' Desk Reference
PDUFA. *See* Prescription Drug User Fee Act
Pediatric dosing, compounded medication for, 75
Pepcid, 164
Percents, conversion of, 176
Personal protective equipment
    aseptic compounding and, 82
    hazardous drugs and, 112
Pestle, compounding and, 68, 76
Pharmacy
    ambulatory, 127
    aseptic IV compounding, 81-83
    automation for, 60-61
    community, 105
    drive-thru window in, 127
    inpatient, 55-61
    Internet, patient protection and, 137-138
    mail order, 46-52
    nuclear, 113
    outsourcing, 105
    satellite, 105
    technology in, 60-61
Pharmacy balance, 65-67
Pharmacy fax form, example of, 26
Pharmacy practice, state regulations and, 140-141
Pharmacy reports, 181-182
Pharmacy software, 16
Pharmacy technician
    Code of Ethics for, 135-136
    math skills for, 183-184
    medication errors reported by, 166
    reference materials for, 171-175
    Spanish for, 127-132
Phenobarbital, 161
Phenytoin, 165
Physical dependency, scheduled drugs and, 159, 160

Physician, name and signature of, medication order and, 56
Physician office, 105
Physicians' Desk Reference, 172, 174
Pints, conversion factors for, 148
Placebo, drug testing and, 151
Plunger, syringe, 98
Polyvinyl chloride, plastic bag made from, 109
Pontocaine, 175
Pounds, conversion of, 147, 177
PPE. *See* Personal protective equipment
Prazosin, 165
Pre-clinical testing, drug approval process and, 150, 151, 157
Prefilter, description of, 90
Prejudice
    communication and, 124-125
    elimination of, 129
Preparation pad, description of, 112
Preparation worksheet, 108
Prescription
    compounded, 75
    conversion of, 184
    data entry for, 17-18
    error in, 167
    home medical equipment and, 31
    inpatient
        medication order and, 56-58
        processing of, 55-59
    interpretation of, 9-12, 169-170
    mail order, 46-52
    patient information for, 19-20, 55, 56
    refilling of, 22-26
        data entry for, 27-29
    rejection of, by insurance company, 185
    retail, processing of, 19-21
Prescription balance, class A, 66-67
Prescription drug discount card, 13
Prescription Drug User Fee Act, 152, 155, 156
Prescription order, 9
    checking of, 20
    filling of, 20
Prevacid, 186
Prilosec, 186
Primary card holder, 14
Prior authorization, 185-189
    home medical equipment and, 31
Prior Authorization Request Form, 185, 188
Privacy rights, 42, 43-44, 45
Procardia, 164
Professional Compounding Centers of America, website of, 71
Professional liability insurance, 139
Progesterone, 186
Propranolol, 165
Protective equipment, aseptic compounding and, 82
Protonix, 186
Proventil, 164
Provigil, 186
Prozac, 164
    lawsuit involving, 136-137
Psychological dependency, scheduled drugs and, 159, 160
Purchase orders, inventory management and, 182
PVC bag, 109

Q

Quarts, conversion factors for, 148

R

Ranitidine, 165
Receiving, of hazardous drugs, 113
Reconstitution, technique for, 105-106
Record keeping, scheduled drugs and, 159
Reference materials, 163, 171-175

Refill, prescription, 22-26
    data entry for, 27-29
Refill request form, example of, 25
Reglan, 164
Reporting
    inventory management and, 181-182
    of medication errors, 166-167
Retail lab, orientation to, 3
Retin-A, 186
Retrovir, 150
Robotics, 60, 61
Roman numerals, conversion of, 177

S

Safety
    drug approval process and, 151, 155
    hazardous drugs and, 112-113
    pharmacy technician ethics and, 135
    for scheduled drugs, 159
Saunders Nursing Drug Handbook, 163
Schedule I drugs, 159
Schedule II drugs, 159
Schedule III drugs, 159
Schedule VI drugs, 159-160
Scheduled drugs, 158-162
Screen tip, definition of, 16
Script. See Prescription
Scruple, conversion factors for, 147
Sea View Hospital Healthcare Museum, website of, 68
Sertraline, 165
Shadowing, definition of, 93
Shaft, syringe, 98
Sharps container, 102, 107
Shipping area, in mail order pharmacy, 47
Shoe covers, aseptic technique and, 87, 88
Side effects, drug testing and, 151, 152
Singulair, 152
Slip-Lok syringe, 82
Soap, antimicrobial, 6
Solu-Cortef, 164
Spanish, common phrases in, for pharmacy technician, 127-132
Spatula
    cleaning of, 7
    compounding and, 68, 72
Spill cleanup, of hazardous drugs, 113
Spill kit, description of, 112
Sporanox, 186
Standard of care, code of ethics and, 136
State pharmacy board, 140
    website for, 22
State regulations, pharmacy practice and, 140-141
Stereotyping, communication and, 124-126
Sterile products, labeling of, 108
Stocking, of hazardous drugs, 113
Storage, of scheduled drugs, 159
Sulfamethoxazole with trimethoprim, 165
Support hose, 32-33
Surgical clinic, 105
Swirling, reconstitution of powder and, 107
Syringe
    Luer-Lok, aseptic compounding and, 82
    parts of, 97, 98
    removing bubbles from, 99
    Slip-Lok, aseptic compounding and, 82
    withdrawing liquid from ampule with, 102-103
Syringe shield, 113

T

Tab key, definition of, 16
Tablespoon, conversion factors for, 148
Tablet/capsule counter, 61
Teaspoon, conversion factors for, 148
Technology, pharmacy, 60-61

Tegretol, 164
Telephone etiquette, 121-122
Temperature, conversion of, 184
Tenormin, 164
Testing, drug approval process and, 150, 157
Text box, definition of, 16
Thermal medication packaging, 61
Timolol, 170
Tip, syringe, 98
Topical tretinoin, 186
Toradol, 164
Torsion balance, 65, 66
Total parenteral nutrition, solution for, 93
TPN. See Total parenteral nutrition
Tray, counting, cleaning of, 7, 8
Tretinoin, 186
Trimethoprim, 165
Tufts Center for the Study of Drug Development, 152
Turnover rate, definition of, 183
Tylenol, 164, 170

U

Unit compliance record, example of, 40
Unit dose, compounding and, 69
Unit dose packaging, 61
United States Pharmacopoeia, Chapter 797, 84, 85, 105
United States Pharmacopoeia Drug Information, 172, 174
University of Arizona College of Pharmacy, website of, 81
User fees, drug approval process and, 155-156
USP. See United States Pharmacopoeia
USP DI. See United States Pharmacopoeia Drug Information

V

Valium, 164
Vertical airflow hood, cleaning of, 95-96
Vertical flow hood, aseptic technique and, 85
Vfend, 186
Viagra, 186
Vial
    aseptic compounding and, 82
    description of, 98
    preparation of, for hazardous drugs, 114
    withdrawing liquid from, 97-100
Vincristine, 165
Visual SuperScript, 16, 181
    refill data entry in, 27-28

W

Walker, fitting patient for, 31
Warfarin, 165
Warning label, 3, 4
Warnings, over-the-counter labeling and, 146
Weighing paper, compounding and, 69
Weight
    conversion factors for, 147
    conversion of, from kilograms to pounds, 177
    patient
        inpatient prescription processing and, 55
        medication order and, 56
Wellbutrin, 164, 186

X

Xanax, 164

Z

Zantac, 164
Zegerid, 186
Zidovudine, 150
Zithromax, 164
Zofran, 164
Zoloft, 164
Zovirax, 164
Zyrtec, 164